DATE DUE			

Exercise
and
Sport Biology

International Series on Sport Sciences, Volume 12

EXERCISE AND SPORT BIOLOGY

Edited by:
Paavo V. Komi, Ph.D.
University of Jyväskylä
Jyväskylä, Finland

Series Editors:
Richard C. Nelson, Ph.D.
and
Chauncey A. Morehouse, Ph.D.
The Pennsylvania State University
University Park, Pennsylvania

Human Kinetics Publishers
Champaign, Illinois

Publications Director: Richard D. Howell

Production Director: Margery Brandfon

Copy Editor: Joyce Mathews

Typesetters: Cathryn Kirkham and Sandra Meier

Text Design and Layout: Denise Peters and Lezli Harris

Proceedings of the International Symposium on Sport Biology held at the Finnish Sports Institute, Vierumäki, Finland, in October 1979.

Volumes 1-11 in this series were published by University Park Press. Volumes 2, 4, 5, 7, 8, 9, 10, 11A, and 11B are available; Volumes 1, 3, and 6 are out of print.

Library of Congress Catalog Card Number: 82-81070

ISBN: 0-931250-29-3

Published by Human Kinetics Publishers, Inc.,
Box 5076, Champaign, Illinois 61820.

CONTENTS

Contributors

H.-J. Appell, Institut für Experimentelle Morphologie, Deutsche Sporthochschule, Carl-Diem-Weg, D-5000 Cologne 41, F.R. Germany

Oded Bar-Or, Department of Research and Sports Medicine, Wingate Institute for Physical Education and Sport, Israel

Tadeusz Bober, Biomechanics Laboratory, Academy of Physical Education, 51-617 Wroclaw, Poland

Carmelo Bosco, Department of Biology of Physical Activity, University of Jyväskylä, SF-40100 Jyväskylä 10, Finland

G. Caldwell, Department of Kinesiology, University of Waterloo, Waterloo, Ontario N2L 3G1, Canada

Wojciech Czajkowski, Academy of Physical Education, Crzegórzecka 24a, Krakow 531-32, Poland

Jachen Denoth, Biomechanics Laboratory, Swiss Federal Institute of Technology, Zurich, Switzerland

Patricio Gatica, Sede Regional del Maule, Pontificia Universidad Católica de Chile, Casilla 617 Talca, Chile

José E. Guajardo, Sede Regional del Maule, Pontificia Universidad Católica de Chile, Casilla 617 Talca, Chile

Mikko Harri, Department of Physiology, University of Kuopio, P.O. Box 138, SF-70101 Kuopio 10, Finland

Eino Heikkinen, Department of Public Health, University of Jyväskylä, SF-40100 Jyväskylä 10, Finland

Eino Hietanen, Department Clinical Physiology, University of Kuopio, Kuopio, Finland

Jussi K. Huttunen, Department of Internal Medicine, University of Kuopio, Kuopio, Finland

Osmo Hänninen, Department of Physiology, University of Kuopio, Kuopio, Finland

Ira Jacobs, Karolinska Institute, S-10401 Stockholm 60, Sweden

Francisco Jara, Sede Regional del Maule, Pontificia Universidad Católica de Chile, Casilla 617 Talca, Chile

Peter Kaiser, Laboratory for Human Performance (FOA 57), Karolinska Hospital, S-10401 Stockholm 60, Sweden

Jan Karlsson, Laboratory for Human Performance (FOA 57), Karolinska Institute, S-10401 Stockholm 60, Sweden

Malgorzata Kolanowska, Department of Bioenergetics, Jędrzej Sniadecki, Academy of Physical Education, 80-336 Gdańsk-Oliwa, Poland

Paavo V. Komi, Department of Biology of Physical Activity, University of Jyväskylä, SF-40100 Jyväskylä 10, Finland

Kati Kukkonen, Department of Physiology, University of Kuopio, Kuopio, Finland

Kornelia Kulig, Biomechanics Laboratory, Academy of Physical Education, 51-617 Wroclaw, Poland

Luis Lara, Sede Regional del Maule, Pontificia Universidad Católica de Chile, Casilla 617 Talca, Chile

Dag Linnarsson, Department of Medical Engineering, Karolinska Institute, S-10401 Stockholm 60, Sweden

Hans Lithell, Department of Geriatrics, University of Uppsala, Box 12042, S-75012 Uppsala 12, Sweden

Domicela Litwińska, Department of Bioenergetics, Jędrzej Sniadecki, Academy of Physical Education, 80-336 Gdańsk-Oliwa, Poland

Esko Länsimies, Department of Clinical Physiology, University of Kuopio, SF-70210 Kuopio 21, Finland

Roberto M. Montecinos, Sede Regional del Maule, Pontificia Universidad Católica de Chile, Casilla 617 Talca, Chile

Robert W. Norman, Department of Kinesiology, University of Waterloo, Waterloo, Ontario N2L 3G1, Canada

Jerzy Popinigis, Department of Bioenergetics, Jędrzej Sniadecki, Academy of Physical Education, 80-336 Gdańsk-Oliwa, Poland

Paavo Rahkila, Department of Biology of Physiology, University of Jyväskylä, SF-40100 Jyväskylä 10, Finland

Rainer Rauramaa, Department of Physiology, University of Kuopio, SF-70210 Kuopio 21, Finland

Klaus Reischle, Institut für Sport und Sportwissenschaft der Universität Heidelberg, Im Neuenheimer Feld 700, 69 Heidelberg, BRD

Heikki Rusko, Department of Biology of Physical Activity, University of Jyväskylä, SF-40100 Jyväskylä 10, Finland

Alicja Rutkowska-Kucharska, Biomechanics Laboratory, Academy of Physical Education, 51-617 Wroclaw, Poland

K. Sahlin, Department of Clinical Chemistry, Serafimer-lasarettet, S-11283 Stockholm, Sweden

Rickard Schéle, Laboratory for Human Performance (FOA 57), Karolinska Institute, S-10401 Stockholm 60, Sweden

Bertil Sjödin, Laboratory for Human Performance (FOA 57), Karolinska Institute, S-10401 Stockholm 60, Sweden

C. Stang-Voss, Institut für Experimentelle Morphologie, Deutsche Sporthochschule, Carl-Diem-Weg, D-5000 Cologne 41, F.R. Germany

Harri Suominen, Department of Public Health, University of Jyväskylä, SF-40100 Jyväskylä 10, Finland

Anna Szczęsna-Kaczmarek, Department of Bioenergetics, Jędrzej Sniadecki, Academy of Physical Education, 80-336 Gdańsk-Oliwa, Poland

Per Tesch, Laboratory for Human Performance (FOA 57), Karolinska Institute, S-10401 Stockholm 60, Sweden

Markku Vainikka, Research Unit for Sport and Physical Fitness, Pitkäkatu 25, SF-40700 Jyväskylä 70, Finland

Jukka T. Viitasalo, Department of Biology of Physical Activity, University of Jyväskylä, SF-40100 Jyväskylä 10, Finland

Erkki Voutilainen, Department of Internal Medicine, University of Kuopio, SF-70210 Kuopio 21, Finland

Takashi Wakabayashi, Department of Pathology, Nagoya City University School of Medicine, Nagoya, Japan

Richard Wallensten, Department of Orthopaedic Surgery, Karolinska Hospital, S-10401 Stockholm 60, Sweden

H.U. Wanner, Swiss Federal Institute of Technology, Department of Physical Education, CH-8092 Zurich, Switzerland

Jakob Waser, Biomechanics Laboratory, Swiss Federal Institute of Technology, CH-8092 Zurich, Switzerland

Preface

This volume, *Exercise and Sport Biology*, includes most of the papers presented at the International Symposium on Sport Biology, which was held in Vierumäki, Finland, October 17 to 19, 1979. The symposium was organized by the Department of Biology of Physical Activity, University of Jyväskylä, in cooperation with the Finnish Society for Research in Sports and Physical Education. In addition to the symposium contributions, the volume also contains other selected original publications related to biology of sport and physical activity.

The most recent data on a variety of topics are reported in this volume, ranging from chapters dealing with basic muscle metabolism to articles of more practical nature of physiology and biomechanics of sport and exercise. "Basic Metabolism and Exercise," "Anaerobic Threshold," "Muscle Fibers, Exercise and Training," "Exercise under Different Environmental Conditions," "Immediate and Training Effects of Endurance Type Exercise," and "Biomechanics of Selected Sports" are the specific chapters within the volume. Most of the authors of the individual contributions are authorities in their specific fields. The editor thanks the authors for their efforts to make their contributions stimulating from both scientific and practical points of view.

The editorial work of this volume was made possible through the financial support from the Ministry of Education, Finland. Special thanks is also extended to my colleagues in the Department of Biology of Physical Activity and to Dr. Jan Karlsson (Karolinska Institute, Stockholm), who was instrumental in recruiting authors for the various contributions.

Paavo V. Komi
Jyväskylä, Finland

Basic Metabolism and Exercise

Effect of Exercise on Intracellular Acid-base Balance in the Skeletal Muscle of Man

K. Sahlin
S:t Eriks sjukhus, Department of Clinical Physiology
Huddinge Sjukhus, Huddinge, Sweden

During strenuous exercise, some energy is provided through the formation of lactic acid, which accumulates in the exercising muscle tissue and blood. As lactic acid at physiological pH values is almost completely dissociated, an equivalent formation of hydrogen ions will occur and cause a decrease in pH.

A change in blood pH will affect the oxygen transport into the cells. Acidosis decreases the affinity of hemoglobin for oxygen (the Bohr effect) and more oxygen can be delivered for a given oxygen tension. It has been calculated that the combined effect of increase in blood temperature (from 37 °C to 39 °C) and decrease in blood pH from 7.4 to 7.2 increases oxygen transfer by about 12% (Astrand and Rodahl, 1970, p.159). A slight extracellular acidosis would thus have a beneficial effect on oxygen transfer and probably also on physical performance.

A decrease in intracellular pH (pH_i) will, however, have a negative effect on energy production within the muscle and on the contraction process. It was therefore suggested many years ago that a decrease in pH_i is the limiting factor for short-term exercise.

Many investigations have been performed to test this hypothesis. Prior to exercise, bicarbonate or ammonium chloride has been administered to produce alkalosis or acidosis, respectively (Asmussen et al., 1948; Denning et al., 1931, 1940; Dill et al., 1932; Dorow et al., 1940; Jones et al., 1977; Kinderman et al., 1977; Margaria et al., 1971; Poulus et al., 1974). In some of the studies maximal physical performances were altered in the expected way, whereas in others no effect was obtained. The conflicting results could be due to the different effects of the pretreatment upon intracellular pH in the working muscles.

Intracellular pH and acid-base balance cannot be derived from extracellular measurements, and to elucidate the role of pH for physical performance, it is necessary to perform intracellular measurements in the exercising muscle.

Changes in Muscle pH during Exercise

Today, it is well known that only minor variations in pH in body fluids are consistent with normal metabolism; however most pH measurement in man has been performed in extracellular fluid. Determination of pH in blood is the most utilized clinical test for acid-base evaluation in patients and has also been used to study acid-base changes during exercise. The determination gives an estimate of extracellular acid-base balance, which in some cases reflects intracellular changes. The hydrogen ion and bicarbonate ion, however, cannot freely pass the cellular membrane and the magnitude of the intracellular acid-base changes therefore cannot be derived from extracellular measurements.

Determinations of pH_i in human skeletal muscle have been performed by: (a) measurements of the degree of dissociation of the weak acids DMO (dimethyloxazolidiene-2.4-dione) or carbonic acid and by (b) electrometric pH measurement in muscle homogenate. In the latter technique, the membrane-surrounded intracellular fluid is mixed with the extracellular fluid. Obtained values will be an average over the muscle sample, where the intracellular compartment will dominate. The pH of resting human muscle was found to be between 6.9 and 7.09 (Table 1), which is in agreement with the majority of animal studies performed.

Measurements after exercise have been performed with the CO_2 technique and the muscle-homogenate technique. The DMO method cannot be used in this situation because the equilibration time takes too long (about 1 hr.). The studies which so far have been performed in human skeletal muscle show that continuous exercise to fatigue decreases muscle pH by 0.5-0.6 units down to a pH of 6.4-6.6 (Table 1), which seems to be the lower limit for physical performance. In a study by Hermansen and Osnes (1972) two subjects performed intermittent bicycle exercise three maximal work bouts of about 1 min. duration to exhaustion with 4 min. rest in between. Blood pH continued to fall during the exercise, whereas muscle pH decreased to about the same level after each exercise bout. This indicated that muscle pH could not decrease further and thus had reached a value where lactic acid production was inhibited.

Table 1—Skeletal Muscle pH at Rest and After Exercise to Fatigue in Man ($\bar{x} \pm SD$)

Method	Muscle pH at rest	Type of exercise	Muscle pH after exercise	Reference
DMO	6.90 ± 0.06 ($n=5$)	—	—	Bittar et al. (1962)
DMO	6.92 ± 0.11 ($n=6$)	—	—	Maschio et al. (1970)
Muscle homogenate	6.92 ± 0.10 ($n=11$)	Running or bicycling to exhaustion. Work time about 2 min.	6.41 ± 0.11 ($n=8$)	Hermansen and Osnes (1972)
Muscle homogenate	7.09 ($n=2$)	Isometric contraction to fatigue. Work time about 45 sec.	6.56 ± 0.07 ($n=8$)	Sahlin et al. (1975)
Muscle homogenate	7.08 ± 0.03 ($n=12$)	Bicycling to exhaustion. Work time 5-10 min.	6.60 ± 0.14 ($n=9$)	Sahlin et al. (1976)
CO_2	7.00 ± 0.06 ($n=13$)	Bicycling to exhaustion. Work time 10-11 min.	6.40 ± 0.1 ($n=6$)	Sahlin et al. (1978a)

Accumulation of Lactic Acid in Muscle
and Blood during Exercise

During exhaustive exercise, hydrogen ions are released within the muscle and pH decreases. As shown in Table 2, the major portion (86-94%) of these hydrogen ions is due to the accumulation of lactic acid, and the remainder is due to accumulation of other acids. If the released H^+ ions were added to an unbuffered solution, the free concentration of H^+ ions would be 31-35 mmol/l and pH would decrease to about 1.5. In muscle, however, pH decreases only to about 6.4-6.6 and the free concentration of H^+ is thus very low. Almost all of the released H^+ ions are taken up by different buffering processes. The extent of pH decreases after the addition of H^+ ions will be determined by the buffering capacity.

Decrease in muscle pH after exercise was found to be linearly related to the muscle content of lactate + pyruvate both after isometric contraction (Figure 1) and after short-term bicycle exercise (Figure 2). These close relationships demonstrate the crucial importance of lactate in the acid-base balance during exercise and raises the question whether muscle lactate can serve as an index for muscle pH. Within the same individual and after short-term continuous exercise, this is probably valid, provided the buffer capacity in muscle is unchanged. The relationship between lactate and muscle pH during intermittent exercise or during long-term exercise is unknown, and pH measurements in muscle must, therefore, be performed in these situations.

During recovery from exhaustive bicycle exercise, lactate content in muscle decreases exponentially (Figure 3). The time taken to decrease lactate to half of the initial value is about 10 min. Some of this lactate is oxidized within the muscle to CO_2 and water; and some is translocated to the blood. In recent studies, evidence has been presented that the muscle is capable of converting lactate to glycogen. Further studies are needed to elucidate this possibility. Recovery in muscle pH has about the same time course as lactate and approaches resting values after 20 min.

During hard exercise, lactate accumulates in the blood. Measurements of the base deficit show that hydrogen ions accumulate in an amount equivalent to lactate during the actual exercise, indicating an equal efflux rate from the muscle (Figure 4). During the first minutes of recovery, base deficit increases more than lactate concentration in the blood, which indicates an efflux of hydrogen ions in excess of lactate during this period. Measurements of pH and acid-base changes in the muscle are in line with these data. The efflux of hydrogen ions in excess of lactate during the early phase of recovery suggests that intermittent exercise has a different lactate-pH relationship than continuous exercise.

Table 2—Accumulation of Acidic Compounds in Muscle During Exercise

	Bicycling to exhaustion (5-10 min.)			Isometric contraction to fatigue (30-50 sec.)		
	mmol/kg dry wt	mmol/kg dry wt		mmol/kg dry wt	mmol H$^+$/kg dry wt	
Lactate	108	108	(a)	85	85	(c)
Pyruvate	0.3	0.3	(a)	2.8	2.8	(c)
Malate	1.5	3	(b)	0.5	1	(d)
Citrate	0	0	(b)	0.5	1.5	(d)
Glucose 6-P	5	2	(b)	15.8	5.8	(c)
Glycerol 1-P	9	2	(b)	8	3.0	(e)

Note. The release of H$^+$ was calculated from the pK$_a$ values and the prevailing muscle pH. (a) Sahlin et al., 1976; (b) Essen, 1978; (c) Ahlborg et al., 1972; (d) Unpublished observations; (e) Bergstrom et al., 1971b.

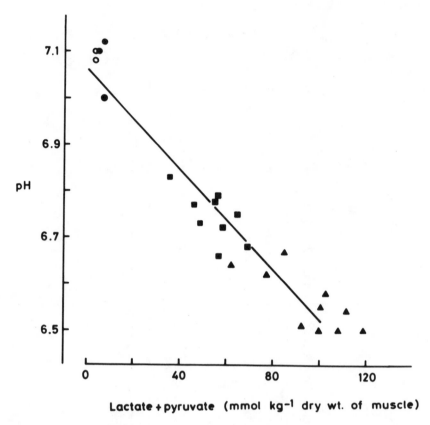

Figure 1—Relationship between pH and content of lactate + pyruvate in muscle biopsies obtained at rest (o), after 15 min., circulatory occlusion (●), after isometric contraction at 68% of the maximum voluntary contraction force sustained for 25 sec. (■) or to fatigue (▲). pH = -0.00532 (lactate + pyruvate) + 7.06; $r = 0.96$; $n = 24$. Reproduced from Sahlin et al. (1975).

Effect of Decreased pH on Intracellular Energy Metabolism in Muscle

A continuous high rate of glycolysis during exercise would result in a severe acidosis in muscle and the whole body. This could affect the homeostasis and the function of acid-labile components or systems in muscle or other more sensitive and critical tissues (i.e., heart and brain). A high concentration of lactate ions in muscle could also be harmful due to the increased osmotic pressure, which would cause a swelling of the muscle. The intracellular water content in muscle has been found to increase during exercise by about 10-20% (Bergstrom et al., 1971a; Sahlin et al., 1978a). A further increase could possibly affect the circulation

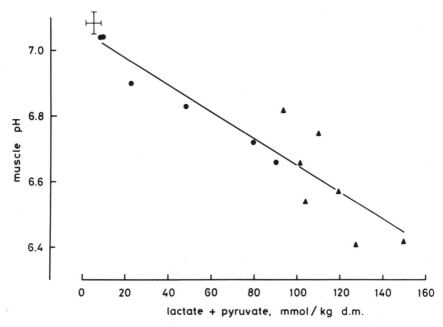

Figure 2—Relationship between pH and content of lactate + pyruvate in muscle samples taken immediately after dynamic exercise. The work was sustained for 5-11 min. at a load of 50-75% (●) and 100% (▲, taken at exhaustion) of W_{max}. pH $= -0.00413$ (lactate + pyruvate) $+ 7.06$; $r = 0.92$; $n = 13$. Reproduced from Sahlin et al. (1976).

within the muscle and cause local ischemia, which would promote anaerobic metabolism with lactate formation.

Numerous investigations have shown that pH affects glycolysis both under aerobic and anaerobic conditions. Alkalosis will thus increase the formation of lactate, whereas acidosis will have an inhibitory effect (for references, see Relman, 1972). The main regulatory step seems to be phosphofructokinase, which exhibits a remarkable pH sensitivity. Other enzymes which are involved in lactic formation and show a decreased activity during acidosis are: adenyl-cyclase, phosphorylase b-kinase, hexokinase and glycerol dehydephosphate-dehydrogenase. The importance of pH for the activity of these enzymes under *in vivo* conditions is not clear.

Investigations by Mitchelson and Hird (1973) and Tobin et al. (1972) into the effect of pH on the mitochondrial function have shown that oxidative phosphorylation is unaffected by the extramitochondrial pH in the range of 6.5-7.0, whereas severe inhibition is noted at pH 6.0 (Mitchelson and Hird, 1973). The absence of physiological carbon dioxide tensions in these experiments, however, makes a translation to an *in vivo* situation difficult. Changes in PCO_2 and HCO_3 might have an effect on

10   Sahlin

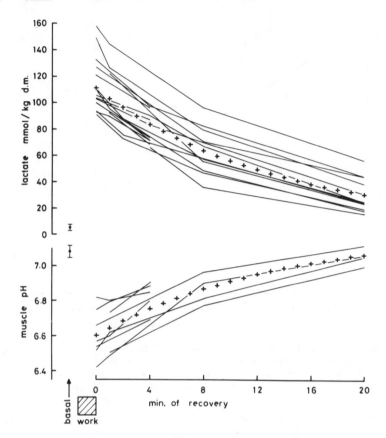

Figure 3—Time course of lactate content and pH in muscle samples taken during recovery from exhaustive dynamic exercise. Work times were between 6 and 11 min. Samples taken in sequence from the same leg have been joined together. Crosses denote the mean curves: lactate $= 5 + 105e^{-0.0733t}$; pH $= 7.19 - 0.584e^{-0.0729t}$ where t denotes minutes of recovery. The equation of the lactate time curve was derived from the mean of semilogarithmic plots of data of each leg. Reproduced from Sahlin et al. (1976).

the citric acid cycle (Adler, 1970) and presence of the CO_2 system could also be a prerequisite for obtaining a pH change within the intramitochondria, when the pH of the surrounding medium is changed. Thus, further experiments are necessary to explore the function of mitochondria at the low pH prevailing after exhaustive exercise.

Muscle contraction is believed to be initiated by a release of Ca^{2+} from the terminal cisterna of the sarcoplasmic reticulum into the cytoplasm. The increase in cytoplasmic Ca^{2+} concentration activates myosin ATPase, which leads to formation of cross-bridges and the breakdown of ATP. The maximum ATPase activity of the actomyosin system in glycerol-extracted muscle fibers was found to be decreased by about 25%

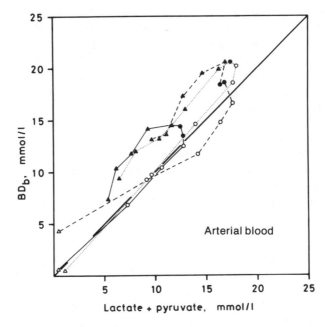

Figure 4—Base deficit in blood (BD_b) compared with content of lactate + pyruvate in blood from arteria brachialis. Samples were taken at rest (Δ), during exercise (o), after 0-2 min. recovery (●), and after 7-30 min. recovery (▲). Values from the same subject are joined together. Content of pyruvate is at all times very small (0.5 mmol/l). Reproduced from Sahlin et al. (1978b).

when pH decreased from 7.0 to 6.5 (Portzehl et al., 1969; Schadler, 1967). In the same studies, it was also found that an increased amount of Ca^{2+} was required to develop 50% of the maximum rate of ATP splitting when pH decreased. In studies on skinned muscle cells, it was found that the maximum tension decreased and the requirement of Ca^{2+} to develop half-maximum tension increased when pH decreased (Donaldson et al., 1978; Fabiato and Fabiato, 1978). This changed requirement for Ca^{2+} during acidosis for developing half-maximum tension was different for various types of muscle. Cardiac muscle was found to be more sensitive than skeletal muscle in this respect (Donaldson et al., 1978; Fabiato and Fabiato, 1978), and it was speculated that this could be one of the reasons for the extreme sensitivity of the cardiac muscle function towards acidosis. In addition to the effect of pH on the contractile proteins, it has been shown that sarcoplasmic reticulum in skeletal muscle binds more Ca during acidosis (Nakamaru and Schwartz, 1972), whereas the SR-system of cardiac muscle does not (Fabiato and Fabiato, 1978). This was thought to accentuate the acidotic sensitivity in cardiac muscle and to diminish it in skeletal muscle.

To further investigate the effect of acidosis on muscle contraction, muscles from rats have been incubated in atmospheres of 5% and 30% CO_2 (which will decrease intracellular pH). We found a decrease in both isometric twitch tension and tetanic tension and a slower relaxation when muscles were incubated in 30% CO_2 (Sahlin, Edström and Sjöholm, unpublished data). Similar changes were obtained when the muscles were stimulated in an anaerobic milieu, during which lactic acid accumulated within the muscle (Sahlin et al., 1981).

The results reviewed in this presentation show that a pronounced acidosis can occur in muscle during short-term exercise and that this acidosis has a negative effect on anaerobic energy production and on the contraction process. Further studies, however, are needed, to assess whether or not intracellular pH is the limiting factor for physical performance.

Acknowledgments

Support from the Swedish Medical Research Council B79-O3X-02647-11B and the Swedish Sports Federation is gratefully acknowledged.

References

Adler, S. 1970. The role of pH, PCO_2 and bicarbonate in regulating rat diaphragm citrate content. *J. Clin. Invest.* **49**:1647-1655.

Ahlborg, B., Bergstrom, J., Ekelund, L.G., Guarnieri, G., Harris, R.C.,Hultman, E., and Nordesjo, L.-O. 1972. Muscle metabolism during isometric exercise performed at constant force. *J. of Appl. Physiol.* **33**:224-228.

Asmussen, E., von Dobeln, W., and Nielsen, M. 1948. Blood lactate and oxygen debt after exhaustive work at different oxygen tensions. *Acta Physiol. Scand.* **15**:57-62.

Astrand, P.O., and Rodahl, K. 1970. *Textbook of Work Physiology.* McGraw-Hill Book Co., New York, NY.

Bergstrom, J., Guarnieri, G., and Hultman, E. 1971a. Carbohydrate metabolism and electrolyte changes in muscle tissue during heavy work. *J. of Appl. Physiol.* **30**:122-125.

Bergstrom, J., Harris, R.C., Hultman, E., and Nordesjo, L.-O. 1971b. Energy-rich phosphagens in dynamic and static work. In: B. Pernow and B. Saltin (eds.) *Advances in Experimental Medicine and Biology,* **11**:341-355, Plenum Press, New York, NY.

Bittar, E.E., Watt, M.F., Pateras, V.R., and Parrish, A.E. 1962. The pH of muscle in Laennec's cirrhosis and uraemia. *Clin. Sci.* **23**:265-276.

Dennig, H., Talbot, J.H., and Dill, D.B. 1931. Effect of acidosis and alkalosis upon capacity for work. *J. of Clin. Invest.* **9**:601-613.

Dennig, H., Becker-Freyseng, H., Rendenbach, H., and Schostak, G. 1940. Leistungssteigerung in lunstlicher Alkalose bei wiederholter Arbeit. (Increased performance in induced alkalosis with repeated work.) *Naunyn-Schmiedebergs Archives for Experimental Pathology and Pharmacology.*

Dill, D.B., Edwards, H.T., and Talbot, J.H. 1932. Alkalosis and the capacity for work. *J. of Biol. Chem.* **97**:1.

Donaldson, S.K.B., Hermansen, L., and Bolles, L. 1978. Differential, direct effects of H^+ on Ca^{2+}-activated force of skinned fibers from the soleus, cardiac, and adductor magnus muscles of rabbits. *Pflugers Archiv.* **376**:55-65.

Dorow, H., Galuba, B., Hellwig, H., and Becker-Freyseng, H. 1940. Der Einfluss kunstlicher Alkalose auf die sportliche Leistung von Laufern und Schwimmern. (The influence of induced alkaloses on the sport performances of runners and swimmers.) *Naunyn Schmiedebergs Archives for Experimental Pathology and Pharmacology.* **195**: 264-266.

Essen, B. 1978. Studies on the regulation of metabolism in human skeletal muscle using intermittent exercise as an experimental model. *Acta Physiol. Scand. Suppl.* **481.**

Fabiato, A., and Fabiato, F. 1978. Effects of pH on the myofilaments and the sarcoplasmic reticulum of skinned cells from cardiac and skeletal muscles. *J. of Physiol.* **276**:233-255.

Hermansen, L., and Osnes, J.-B. 1972. Blood and muscle pH after maximal exercise in man. *J. of Appl. Physiol.* **32**:304-308.

Jones, N.L., Sutton, J.R., Taylor, R., and Toews, C.J. Effect of pH on cardiorespiratory and metabolic responses to exercise. *J. of Appl. Physiol.* **43**:959-964.

Kindermann, W., Keul, J. and Huber, G. 1977. Physical exercise after induced alkalosis (bicarbonate or tris buffer). *Europ. J. of Appl. Physiol. and Occup. Physiol.* **37**:197-204.

Margaria, R., Aghemo, P., and Sassi, G. 1971. Effect of alkalosis on performance and lactate formation in supramaximal exercise. Int. Z. agnewe. Physiol. **29**:215-223.

Maschio, G., Bazzato, G., Bertoglia, E., Sardini, D., Mioni, G., D'Angelo, A., and Marzo, A. 1970. Intracellular pH and electrolyte content of skeletal muscle in patients with chronic renal acidosis. *Nephron.* **7**:481-487.

Mitchelson, K.R., and Hird, F.J.R. 1973. Effect of pH and halothane on muscle and liver mitochondria. *Am. J. Physiol.* **225**:1393-1398.

Nakamaru, Y., and Schwartz, A. 1973. The influence of hydrogen ion concentration on calcium binding and release by skeletal muscle sarcoplasmic reticulum. *J. Gen. Physiol.* **59**:22-32.

Portzehl, H., Zaoralek, P., and Gaudin, J. 1969. The activation by $Ca^{2\pm}$ of the ATPase of extracted muscle fibrils with variation of ionic strength, pH, and concentration of MgATP. *Biochim. Biophys. Acta.* **189**:440-448.

Poulus, A.J., Docter, H.J., and Westra, H.G. 1924. Acid-base balance and subjective feelings of fatigue during physical exercise. *Europ. J. of Appl. Physiol. and Occup. Physiol.* **33**:207-213.

Relman, A.S. 1966. The participation of cells in disturbances of acid-base balance. *Annals of the New York Academy of Sciences.* **133**:160-170.

Sahlin, K., Alvestrand, A., Brandt, R., and Hultman, E. 1978a. Intra-cellular pH and bicarbonate concentration in human muscle during recovery from exercise. *J. of Appl. Physiol.* **45**:474-480.

Sahlin, K., Alvestrand, A., Brandt, R., and Hultman, E. 1978b. Acid-base balance in blood during exhaustive exercise and the following recovery period. *Acta Physiol. Scand.* **104**:370-372.

Sahlin, K., Edstrom, L., Sjöholm, H., and Hultman, E. 1981. Effects of lactic acid accumulation and ATP decrease on muscle tension and relaxation. *Am. J. Physiol.* **240**:C121-C126.

Sahlin, K., Harris, R.C., and Hultman, E. 1975. Creatine kinase equilibrium and lactate content compared with muscle pH in tissue samples obtained after isometric exercise. *Biochem. J.* **152**:73-180.

Sahlin, K., Harris, R.C., Nylind, B., and Hultman, E. 1976. Lactate content and pH in muscle samples obtained after dynamic exercise. *Pflugers Archiv.* **367**:143-149.

Schadler, M. 1967. *Proportionale Aktiverung von ATPase-Aktivitat und Kontraktionsspannung durch Calciumionen in isolierten contractilen Strukturen verschiedener Muskelarten.*(Proportional activation from ATPase activity and tension of contraction through calcium loss in isolated contracile structures of various species of muscles.)

Tobin, R.B., Macherer, C.R., and Mehlman, M.A. 1972. pH effects of oxidative phosphorylation of rat liver mitochondria. *Am. J. Physiol.***223**:83-83.

Oxidative Phosphorylation
Under Extreme Acidic Conditions

Jerzy Popinigis, Magorzata Kolanowska,
Anna Szczesna-Kaczmarek, Domicela Litwinska,
and **Takashi Wakabayashi**
Academy of Physical Education, Poland

The adenosine triphosphate (ATP) required for any exercise can be supplied in two ways:

I. Transfer of High Energy
Phosphate from Phosphocreatine (CP) to
Adenosine Diphosphate (ADP)

This is a very fast reaction which replenishes intracellular ATP. The reaction is catalyzed by creatine phosphokinase, an enzyme which is present in both extramitochondrial and intramitochondrial compartments (Jacobs et al., 1964). The latter isoenzyme is coupled to ATP-ADP translocase (Saks et al., 1977).

II. Phosphorylation of ADP

Because the historically warranted names "aerobic" and "anaerobic" are misleading (Holloszy, 1975), these terms have been replaced here with "intramitochondrial" and "extramitochondrial" modes of ATP formation, respectively.

IIa. Intramitochondrial ADP Phosphorylation

The energy required for ATP formation is mainly provided by the respiratory chain. The process is called "oxidative phosphorylation." Oxygen availability is an absolute requirement for this mode of ATP formation. The single substrate-level phosphorylation (which occurs intramitochondrially even under anaerobic conditions) plays no significant role in providing ATP for muscular work.

It is now generally accepted that fatty acids are quantitatively the most important substrate for the IIa system in skeletal muscle in various metabolic states (Costill et al., 1977; Rennie et al., 1976). Other substrates of practical significance are malate, pyruvate, ketone bodies, and glycerolphosphate. The rate of respiration is accelerated by ADP (state 4 to state 3 transition; Chance and Williams, 1956), regulated by ATP/ADP ratio (Bohnensack and Kunz, 1978; Davis and Lumeng, 1975), and the rate-limiting step is the activity of adenine nucleotide translocase (Davis and Lumeng, 1975). The reported K_m for this enzyme is 13 mu (Davis and Lumeng, 1975). This is a very efficient mode of ATP production, but because of its low speed (the time required for oxygen, substrates, ADP, and phosphate transport into the mitochondria), the II system is used mainly when exercise is of low power output and long duration (Fox, 1977).

Endurance training increases the capacity of the IIa system through an increase in the levels of a number of mitochondrial enzymes (for review, see Holloszy, 1975). The same effect on aerobic power was seen after interval training (Fox, 1977).

IIb. Extramitochondrial ADP Phosphorylation

Although this system has traditionally been named "anaerobic," it is also active in the presence of oxygen. Two enzymes, phosphoglycerate kinase and pyruvate kinase with K_m for ADP 300 and 350 mu, respectively, catalyze transfer of high energy phosphate from 1, 3 diphosphoglycerate (1, 3 DPG) and phosphoenolopyruvate (PEP) to ADP, respectively, for formation of ATP. The process is called "substrate-level phosphorylation." The 1, 3 DPG and PEP are "high energy" metabolites, the formation of which occur through the metabolism of glycogen or glucose to lactate (glycolysis) or pyruvate (glycolytic pathway). The speed of the IIb system is controlled by ATP/ADP ratio, as well as influenced by NADH/NAD. The rate of this metabolism is facilitated by cAMP (at the level of glycogen phosphorylase) and inhibited by ATP, CP, and citrate (at the level of phosphofructokinase). The IIb system provides energy for muscular work of high intensity and when greater power is needed (Fox, 1977).

The capacity of the II system increases after sprint training. The effect is rationalized assuming that the trained muscle utilizes ATP and CP stores faster and removes the course-limiting of glycolysis more quickly

(Rehunen et al., 1976).

The extent to which systems IIa and IIb provide energy for working muscle is determined mainly by the intensity of exercise. At rest and during light or moderate exercise, system IIa almost completely fulfills the energy requirement through fatty acid oxidation (Rosell and Saltin, 1973). But when the intensity of exercise becomes higher than 60% of VO_2 max there is a sudden general switch of metabolism. The role of the IIa system becomes replaced by system IIb in energy production. Up till now, no reasonable explanation has been given for this phenomenon. Because piridine nucleotides in the respiratory chain of mitochondria are, in these conditions, in an oxidized state (Jobsis and Stainsby, 1968), it is known that this general switch in the mode of ATP formation cannot be attributed to hypoxia (Edington et al., 1973). The most probable explanation, therefore, is that of Jobsis and Stainsby (1968), who suggested that the IIa to IIb transition is caused by a decrease of pyruvate utilization in the citrate cycle.

This problem was reexamined in this investigation. The experiments were performed with mitochondria isolated from the skeletal muscle of the rat. In order to simulate an *in vivo* situation under rest and heavy exercise, the media of pH of 7.0 and 6.4, respectively, were used after Sahlin et al. (1978), incorporating also their observation that at pH 7.0 the intracellular HCO_3 concentration is about 10 mM. In our experiments, other very important information was also used to show that when the muscle mitochondria are incubated with ATP and HCO_3, the rate of pyruvate oxidation is the same as in the presence of malate (J.E. Davis, personal communication). Moreover, this respiration is very sensitive to ATP/ADP ratio and decreases when ADP concentration in the incubation medium is increased. Undoubtedly, because pyruvate carbosylase activity in muscle mitochondria is considered to be low, Davis' finding is of great importance, especially for sport biochemistry. It is our contention that this provides a very rational explanation for the IIa to IIb switch of energy metabolism with an increasing work load. Based on Davis' observation, experimental conditions were set up in which palmitylocarnitine was oxidized in the absence of added malate. It was shown that this coupled to ATP synthesis respiration required pyruvate HCO_3 and ATP. In the absence of HCO_3 and in the presence of ADP, the palmitylocarnitine oxidation was strictly dependent on the presence of malate. Discussion of the significance of the observations for the IIa to IIb metabolic transition follows.

Materials and Methods

Muscle mitochondria from the skeletal muscle of the rat's hind legs

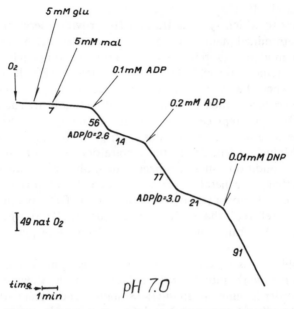

Figure 1—Oxidation of glutamate plus malate in skeletal muscle mitochondria of rat at pH 7.0. The amount of added mitochondria corresponded to 0.45 mg of protein. Other additions as indicated in the figure. For experimental conditions, see Materials and Methods. The rate of respiration is expressed as a natams $O_2 \times$ min.$^{-1}$. Abbreviations: glutamate (glu), malate (mal) adeonosine diphosphate (ADP), 2,4-dinitrophenol (DNP).

were isolated in the cold according to the method of Swierczynski et al. (1975).

Oxygen uptake was measured polarographically with a Clark oxygen electrode (Gilson Polarograph) in 2-ml cells, employing media of pH 6.4 and of pH 7.0. Each medium contained 50 mM Pipes-KOH, 15 mM KCl, 5 mM buffer phosphate, 6 mM EDTA, 0.2% bovine serum albumin (BSA) free from fatty acids, 1.25 mM $MgCl_2$, and 0.0025 mM cytochrome c.

Adrenal cortex mitochondria of swine were isolated according to the method of Allmann et al. (1970). The rate of oxygen consumption was measured with a Clark-type electrode (Gilson Polarograph) in a medium of pH 6.1, which contained 50 mM Trizma-HCl, 15 mM KCl, 5 mM buffer phosphate, and 2 mM EDTA.

The mitochondrial protein concentrations were assayed according to Lowry et al. (1951) with bovine serum as a standard.

Results

Neither the glutamate plus malate nor palmitylocarnitine plus malate

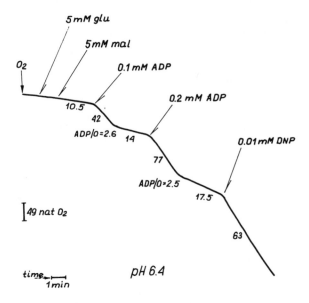

Figure 2—Oxidation of glutamate plus malate in skeletal muscle mitocnondria of rat at pH 6.4. The experimental conditions were the same as in Figure 1 except that pH 6.4 medium was employed. For abbreviations, see Figure 1.

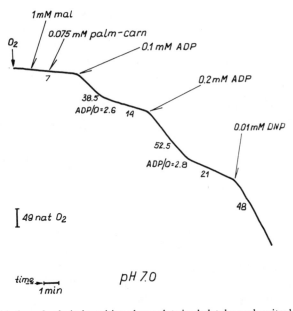

Figure 3—Oxidation of palmitylcarnitine plus malate in skeletal muscle mitochondria of rat at pH 7.0. Experimental conditions and the amount of mitochondria used were the same as in Figure 1. Abbreviations: palmitylcarnitine (palm – carn), for the others, see Figure 1.

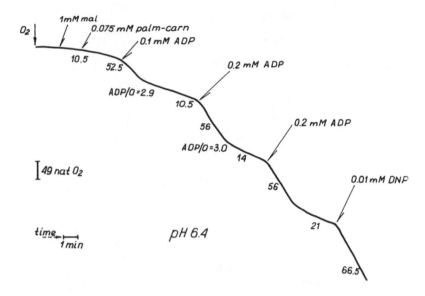

Figure 4—Oxidation of palmitylcarnitine plus malate in skeletal muscle mitochondria of rat at pH 6.4. Experimental conditions and the amount of mitochondria were the same as in Figure 1, except that pH 6.4 medium was employed. Abbreviations as in Figures 1 and 3.

oxidation in rat skeletal muscle mitochondria was affected by the drop in pH value from 7.0 to 6.4. This is indicated in the results presented in Figures 1-4. It can be seen that glutamate plus malate oxidation was well coupled at pH 7.0 (Figure 1), and when the same experiment was repeated at pH 6.4, the ADP/O ratio was still above 2.5 (Figure 2.) Similar results were also seen with palmitylocarnitine plus malate as a substrate. Mitochondria were well coupled in both pH 7.0 (Figure 3) as well as pH 6.4 media (Figure 4). At pH as low as 6.1, mitochondria isolated from adrenal cortex of swine also showed a very high degree of coupling (Figure 5). Moreover, the rate of state 4 succinate oxidation was also increased by deoxycorticosterone (DOC). This indicates that adrenal mitochondria can perform DOC to corticosterone 11-hydroxylation under extreme acidic conditions.

The aim of the experiment presented in Figure 6 was to simulate conditions which are supposed to be present in skeletal muscle at rest. Pyruvate, 10 mM HCO_3 and ATP were first added to the mitochondria. This was followed by palmitylocarnitine and additions of ADP induced state 4 to state 3 transition with ADP/O ratio of 2.2 and 2.3. To simulate conditions which are supposed to be present during conditions of extreme exercise, in the next experiment (Figure 7) the pH of the medium was changed to 6.4, HCO_3 was omitted, and ATP was replaced by ADP.

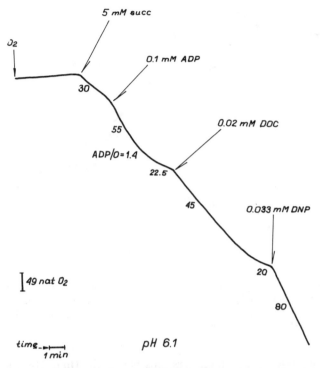

Figure 5—Oxidative phosphorylation and 11 β-hydroxylation in adrenal cortex mitochondria of swine at pH 6.1. For experimental conditions, see Materials and Methods. Abbreviations: succinate (succ), deoxycorticosterone (DOC). The amount of mitochondria added correspond to 3.5 mg of protein.

Under such conditions, the rate of pyruvate plus palmitylocarnitine oxidation was negligible and did not increase after ADP.

Discussion

The aim of this investigation was to elucidate factors responsible for IIa to IIb transition. Because previous observations (Brucker et al., 1972; Popinigis et al., 1971) revealed that an increase in H^+ concentration exerted a profound effect on metabolism and ultrastructure of liver mitochondria, first an attempt was made to examine effects of pH on oxidative phosphorylation in mitochondria isolated from skeletal muscle of rats. It was demonstrated that both malate plus glutamate as well as palmitylocarnitine plus malate oxidations were well coupled to ATP synthesis in a pH 6.4 medium. This indicated that the drop in pH cannot be

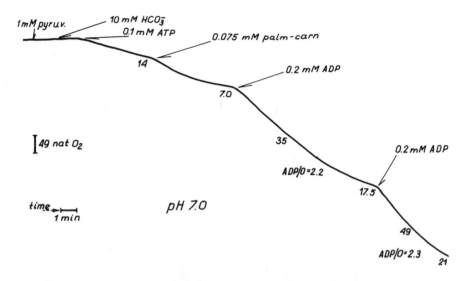

Figure 6—The pyruvate plus $NaHCO_3$ plus ATP-dependent palmitylcarnitine oxidation in skeletal muscle mitochondria of rat at pH 7.0. Experimental conditions and the amount of mitochondria were the same as in Figure 1. Abbreviations: pyruvate (pyruv.), adenosine triphosphate (ATP), others as in previous figures.

considered as a primary factor responsible for the IIa to IIb transition. In addition, it was observed that in mitochondria isolated from the adrenal cortex of swine, neither oxidative phosphorylation nor 11-β-hydroxylation is impaired by a low (6.1) pH of the medium. It has been reported (Kolanowska et al., 1979) that only under acidic conditions can these mitochondria carry out oxidative phosphorylation after 11-β-hydroxylation ceases. On the basis of experimental results shown in Figures 6 and 7, the following explanation for the IIa → IIb transition is presented.

At rest and during relatively moderate muscular activity (low ATP-ase load of Dynnik, 1979), energy is provided through the IIa system by fatty acid oxidation. The rate of this respiration is limited by the supply of acetylCoA acceptor (oxaloacetate- OAA), which is presumably formed by carboxylation of pyruvate. The rather high ATP/ADP ratio and presence of HCO_3 meets these requirements. With higher work loads (higher ATP-ase load), the IIa system is still functional despite the stimulation of glycolysis. But, because of the low ATP/ADP ratio and decrease in HCO_3 concentration, OAA is not formed from pyruvate and, thus, fatty acid oxidation ceases. The rate of mitochondrial respiration becomes dependent on the supply of reducing equivalents from cytoplasm via the malate-aspartate shuttle (Edington et al., 1973). Digerness and Reddy (1976), studying the malate-asparate shuttle in heart mitochondria, have found that, in the presence of pyruvate,

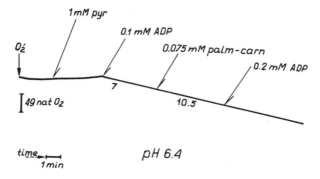

Figure 7—The inability of skeletal muscle mitochondria to oxidize palmitylcarnitine plus pyruvate in the absence of ATP and NaHCHO₃. Experimental conditions were the same as in Figure 6 except that pH medium was 6.4.

glutamate, and ADP, isolated heart mitochondria incorporate all malate into asparate—which leaves the mitochondria. We believe that after IIa to IIb transition, malate cannot act as the acetylCoA acceptor required for palmitylocarnitine oxidation, because glutamate concentration during prolonged muscle stimulation decreases (Edington et al., 1973). One may postulate that after fatty acid oxidation ceases, the respiratory chain utilizes reducing equivalents delivered from cytoplasm by the malate-asparate shuttle. Several authors have suggested the role played by hydrogen shuttles in lowering lactate production during exercise (for review, see Holloszy, 1975). Increases in the cytoplasmic levels of aspartate and in extramitochondrial H^+ concentration may limit reducing equivalent import and, therefore, slowing down the rate of respiration by influencing activity of the glutamate translocator (LaNoue and Duszynski, 1978). If it is assumed that IIa to IIb transition is reversible, i.e., during recovery from exercise, the ATP/ADP ratio and bicarbonate concentration increase again, it provides an explanation of why during vigorous work, the muscle produces lactate and why, during recovery and light work (30-40% of VO_2 max), it removes the lactate from the blood (Stamford et al., 1978).

At present, the possibility cannot be ruled out that under *in vivo* conditions other factors are also involved. For example, the regulatory role played by the ultrastructure of mitochondria in metabolism was pointed out recently (Popinigis, 1978). It is known that upon acidification, the mitochondria maintain or even increase their ability to accumulate calcium (Pearson et al., 1977). Ultrastructural transitions of mitochondria can therefore be predicted. In our experimental conditions the structural rearrangements were prevented using calcium chelator EDTA.

References

Allmann, D.W., Wakabayashi, T., Korman, E.F., and Green, D.E. 1970. Studies on the transition of the cristal membrane from the orthodox to the aggregated configuration. I: Topology of bovine adrenal mitochondria in the orthodox configuration. *Bioenergetics* 1:73-86.

Bohnensack, R., and Kunz, W., 1978. Mathematical model of regulation of oxidative phosphorylation in intact mitochondria. *Acta Biol. Med. Germ.* 37:97-112.

Brucker, R.F., Williams, C.H., Popinigis, J., Galvez, T.L., Vail, W.J., and Taylor, C.A. 1972. In vitro studies on liver mitochondria and skeletal muscle sarcoplasmic reticulum fragments isolated from hyperpyrexic swine. In: B.A. Britt, R. A. Gordon, and W. Kalow (eds.). *Proceedings of 1st International Symposium on Malignant Hyperthermia*, pp. 238-270. Charles Thomas, Springfield, IL.

Chance, B. and Williams, G.R. 1956. The respiratory chain and oxidative phosphorylation. *Advan. Enzymol.* 17:65-134.

Costill, D.L., Coyle, E., Dalsky, G., Evans, W., Fink, W., and Hoopes, D. 1977. Effects of elevated plasma FFA and insulin on muscle glycogen usage during exercise. *J. Appl. Physiol. Respirat. Environ. Exercise Physiol.* 43(4):695-699.

Davis, E.J., and Lumeng, L. 1975. Relationships between the phosphorylation potentials generated by liver mitochondria and respiratory rate under conditions of adenosine diphosphate control. *J. Biol. Chem.* 250:2275-2282.

Digerness, S.B., and Reddy, W.J. 1976. The malate-asparate shuttle in heart mitochondria. *J. Mol. Cel. Cardiol.* 8:779-785.

Dynnik, V.V. 1979. Theoretical studies on the mechanism of the interaction between glycogenolysis, tricarboxylic acid cycle, H-transferring shuttles and β-oxidation. *Abstracts of the 8th International Colloquium on Bioenergetics and Mitochondria:* **26.**

Edington, D.W., Ward, G.R., Saville, W.A. 1973. Energy metabolism of working muscle: Concentration profiles of selected metabolites. *Am. J. Physiol.* 224:1375-1380.

Fox, E.L. 1977. Physical training: Methods and effects. *Orthop. Clin. North Am.* 8:533-548.

Holloszy, J.O. 1975. Adaptation of skeletal muscle to endurance exercise. *Med. Sci. Sport* 7:155-164.

Jacobs, H., Heldt, H.W., and Klingenberg, M. 1964. High activity of creatine kinase in mitochondria from muscle and brain and evidence for a separate mitochondrial isoenzyme of creatine kinase. *Biochim. Biophys. Res. Comm.* 16:516-521.

Jobsis, F.F. and Stainsby, W.N. 1968. Oxidation of NADH during contractions of circulated mammalian skeletal muscle. *Resp. Physiol.* 4:292-300.

Kolanowska, M., Szczesna-Kaczmarek, A., Litwinska, D., and Popinigis, J. 1979. Possible role of extramitochondrial pH in regulation of oxidative phosphorylation and 11-β-hydroxylation in adrenal mitochondria. *Abstracts of the 8th International Colloquium on Bioenergetics and Mitochondria.* **70.**

LaNoue, K. and Duszynski, J. 1978. The influence of protons on the glutamate-aspartate carrier in the mitochondrial membrane. In: Azzone, G.F. et al. (eds.) *The Proton and Calcium Pumps,* pp.297-307. Elsevier North-Holland Biomedical Press, Amsterdam.

Lowry, O.H., Rosebrough, N.J., Farr, A.L., and Randall, R.J. 1951. Protein measurement with the folin phenol reagent. *J. Biol. Chem.* **193**:265-275.

Pearson, A.M., Kanda, T., Cornforth, D.P., Merkel, R.A., and Porzio, M.A. 1977. Effects of pH and temperature on calcium uptake and release by sarcoplasmic reticulum. *Meat Sci.* **1**:155-165.

Popinigis, J. 1978. Permeability of membrane as a factor determining the rate of mitochondrial respiration: Role of ultrastructure. In: Sidney Fleischer, Youssef Hatefi, David H. MacLennan, and Alexander Tzagoloff (eds.). *The Molecular Biology of Membranes,* pp.75-101. Plenum Publishing Corporation, NY.

Popinigis, J., Takahashi, Y., Wakabayashi, T., Hull, R. M., and Willams, C.H. 1971. Some aspects of mitochondrial structure. *FEBS Letters* **19**:221-224.

Rehunen, S., Naveri, H., Kuoppasalmi, K., Tulikoura, I, and Harkonen, I. 1976. Regulation of muscle metabolism during short-term physical exercise. *Sport Wyczynowy.* **11**:21-26.

Rennie, M., Winder, W.M., and Holloszy, 1976. A sparing effect of increased free fatty acids on muscle glycogen content in exercising rat. *Biochem. J.* **156**:647-655.

Rosell, S., and Saltin, B. 1973. Energy need, delivery, and utilization in muscular exercise. In: Geoffrey H. Bourne (ed.), *The Structure and Function of Muscle* (2nd ed.). Vol. 3, pp.185-221. Academic Press, Inc., New York and London.

Sahlin, K., Alvestrand, A., Brandt, R., and Hultman, E. 1978. Intracellular pH and bicarbonate concentration in human muscle during recovery from exercise. *J. Appl. Physiol. Respirat. Environ. Exercise Physiol.* **45**:474-480.

Saks, V.A., Seppet, E.K., and Lyulina, N.V. 1977. Comparative investigation of the role of creatine phosphokinase isoenzymes in energy metabolism of skeletal muscles and myocardium. *Biokhimiya* **42**:579-588 (in Russian), English version pp. 445-452.

Swierczynski, J., Aleksandrowicz, Z., and Zydowo, M. 1975. Effect of some steroids and α-tocopherol on cytochrome c-induced extramitochondrial NADH oxidation by human and rat skeletal muscle mitochondria. *Int. J. Biochem.* **6**:757-763.

Some Factors Determining the Lipoprotein-Lipase Activity of Skeletal Muscle During Heavy Exercise

Hans Lithell
University of Uppsala, Sweden

Jan Karlsson
Karolinska Institute, Sweden

Neutral fat in the diet is taken up in the intestine after hydrolysis by pancreatic lipase. In the intestinal wall, the fatty acids are utilized for the resynthesis of triglycerides, which are incorporated into large macromolecules or chylomicrons (Brunzell et al., 1978). The chylomicrons are introduced into the blood plasma via the lymphatics, where the triglyceride content is rapidly diminished through a lipolytic process mediated by the enzyme lipoprotein lipase (LPL) (Brunzell et al., 1978). During the day, lipolysis of triglycerides stored in the adipose tissue is continuous, with liberation of fatty acids into the circulation (Brunzell et al., 1978). A portion of these fatty acids is processed by the liver, where it is used for the synthesis of triglycerides, which are incorporated into very low density lipoproteins (Brunzell et al., 1978). The triglycerides in chylomicrons and very low density lipoproteins are metabolized by the same metabolic pathway (Brunzell et al., 1978). In the fed state, however, most of the triglycerides are taken up by adipose tissue, whereas in the fasting state, as much as 48% of the circulating triglycerides are taken up by skeletal muscle tissue (Rossner, 1974). The different distributions of the triglycerides in the fasting and in the fed states are probably effected by different degrees of activity of the LPL in the two tissues. It has been shown (Lithell et al., 1978) that in human skeletal muscle the activity of LPL is greater in the fasting state in the morning than in the fed state in the afternoon (Figure 1) and the reverse pattern is found in adipose tissue (Figure 2).

It has been shown by others that well-trained people have a relatively larger combustion of fat than untrained people (Hermansen et al., 1967).

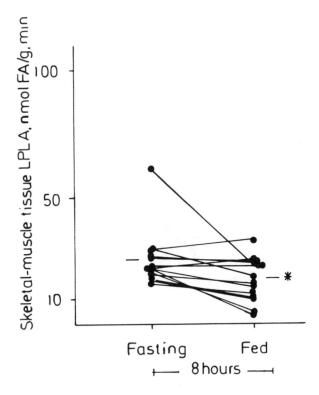

Figure 1—Lipoprotein-lipase activity (LPLA) of skeletal muscle tissue (nmol fatty acid (FA) $\times$ g^{-1} $\times$ min^{-1}) in the fasting state in the morning and after meals 8 hr. later in 15 healthy medical students. $p < 0.05$ when tested by Student's paired t-test.

During prolonged exercise, the metabolism is diverted towards a larger fat combustion (Hermansen et al., 1967). The increased use of fatty acids during exercise can only be partially accounted for by an increased uptake of free fatty acids from the blood circulation. That means that the rest of the fatty acids that are being utilized in combustion must be derived from triglycerides. Two principal stores of triglycerides are available for the working skeletal muscle. One is the small, fat droplets, located in the myofibrils, that can be quantified by chemical analysis or electron microscopic determinations and the other is the circulating triglycerides in very low density lipoproteins (or chylomicrons). Great technological and methodological problems are involved in quantifying the uptake of triglycerides from the circulation by measurements of the arteriovenous differences. As it is known from studies of experiments on animals that the uptake of triglycerides in muscle tissue is directly related to the heparin-releasable LPL (Linder et al., 1976), lipoprotein-lipase activity (LPLA) was used as an indicator of the uptake of triglycerides in

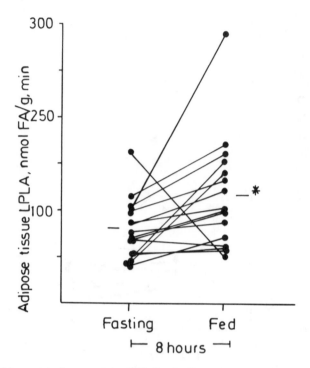

Figure 2—Lipoprotein-lipase activity (LPLA) of adipose tissue (nmol fatty acid (FA) ×
g⁻¹ × min) in the fasting state in the morning and after several meals 8 hr. later. Statistics
as in Figure 1.

different tissues. To quantify LPLA, a reaction medium is used, in which
an artificial triglyceride/phospholipid emulsion is activated by the addition of serum. Heparin is included in the reaction medium, thereby
liberating the functional LPL from its site on the endothelial lining of
capillaries and small blood vessels (Lithell and Boberg, 1978).

In the rat, short, heavy physical work changes the pattern seen in the
fed state with a low LPLA in skeletal muscle and a high degree of activity
in adipose tissue towards the pattern normally found in the fasting state,
i.e., a high LPLA in muscle tissue and a low degree of activity in adipose
tissue (Nikkilä et al., 1963). A similar study was made of healthy, medical students, who exercised on a bicycle ergometer for 1 hr. (Lithell et al.,
1979). The working load was set so that they were exhausted towards the
end of the work. During this short-term physical activity, there was no
reversion to the LPLA pattern of the fed state. On the contrary, in
adipose tissue, a further significant increase of the LPLA occurred,
probably a later response to the meals of the earlier part of the day.

More prolonged physical exercise yields a different result (Lithell et

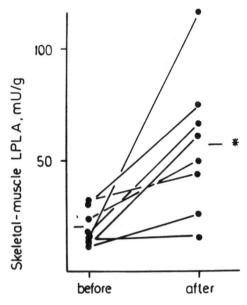

Figure 3—Lipoprotein-lipase activity (LPLA) of skeletal muscle mU/g (1 mU = 1 mol fatty acid released per min.), before and after an 85-km skiing race in eight subjects. (One did not complete the race.) Statistics as in Figure 1.

al., 1979). As shown in Figure 3, the LPLA in skeletal muscle increased significantly in a group of seven subjects who took part in a 85-km skiing race. The variation within the group in which some individuals did not increase their LPLA, in contrast to others who increased it five- to six-fold, was found to be related to their degree of physical fitness. As shown in Figure 4, a significant relationship existed between the prerace training distance covered by the individual and the increase in LPLA during the race. A similar relationship was found between the maximal oxygen uptake and the increase of LPLA (Figure 5). These relationships indicate that individuals who were well trained did not have a "need" for a further increase of their LPLA. This may be explained by the findings of the changes in the lipid droplets in the cells that were studied in skeletal muscle biopsies taken on the same occasion from these individuals. As shown in Figure 6, those individuals who had trained most before the race had the largest stores of neutral fat in the muscle cells. There was a very close correlation between the maximal oxygen uptake per kilogram of body weight and the decrease of lipid droplets during the race (Figure 7). This means that those who were best trained had the largest stores of lipid in their cells and used more of these stores than those who were less well trained. An inverse relationship also existed between the amount of neutral fat in the cells before the race and the in-

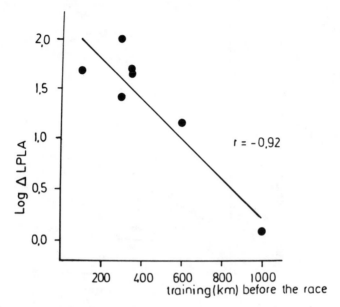

Figure 4—Relationship between the prerace training distance (km) and the change of lipoprotein-lipase activity (LPLA) during the race in seven subjects. $r = 0.92, p < 0.001$ indicates the degree of significance of the r-value calculated by the method of least squares.

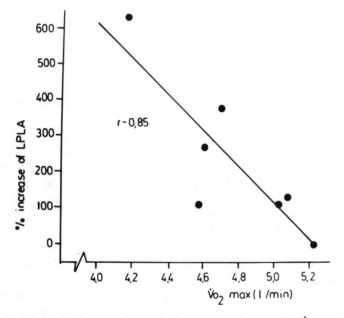

Figure 5—Relationship between the maximal oxygen uptake capacity ($\dot{V}_{O_2}$max) (1/min) determined before the race and the percentage of increase in lipoprotein-lipase activity (LPLA) during the race. $r = 0.85$, $p < 0.01$. Statistics as in Figure 4.

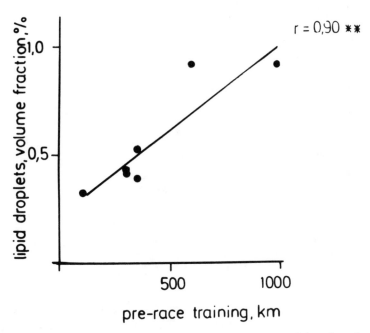

Figure 6—Relationship between the prerace training distance (km) and the volume fraction (%) of lipid droplets in the myofibrils before the race. $r = 0.90$, $p < 0.01$. Statistics as in Figure 4.

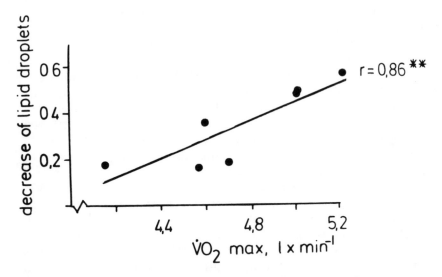

Figure 7—Relationship between the maximal oxygen uptake capacity ($\dot{V}_{O_2}$max) (1/min) and the decrease of lipid droplets in the myofibrils during the race. $r = 0.86$, $p < 0.01$. Statistics as in Figure 4.

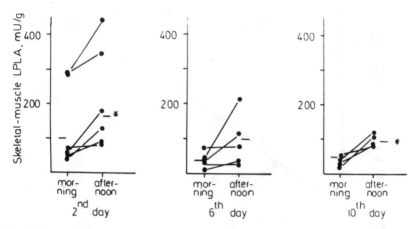

Figure 8—Lipoprotein-lipase activity (LPLA) of skeletal muscle tissue in the morning and in the afternoon of days of heavy work (Days 2 and 10) and medium-heavy work (Day 6) in six soldiers on a 10-day march. Statistics as in Figure 1.

crease of LPLA during the race, so that those who had the largest stores of lipid had no increase in their LPLA during the race. These findings can be interpreted by saying that a trained individual has larger stores of lipids in the cells and uses these stores before any change occurs in his ability to take up neutral fat from circulating lipoproteins. This hypothesis also gives a possible explanation for the delayed increase of LPLA in well-trained subjects, for it has been suggested that high levels of intracellular fatty acids inhibit the synthesis of LPL (Pykalisto, 1970). A high level of fatty acids is probably present in the cells during the lipolysis of the neutral fat.

These findings then raise the question of whether well-trained subjects ever have any change in the level of LPLA in their skeletal muscle. This has been studied in a group of Swedish soldiers, who performed very strenuous work for 10 days (Lithell et al., 1981). Morning and afternoon specimens of skeletal muscle tissue were taken and analyzed for LPLA. Despite the intake of several meals during the day, heavy physical work for 8 to 9 hr. was followed by a significant increase of LPLA in skeletal muscle tissue in all subjects during the days with the heaviest work, whereas, during the day with a workload of intermediate intensity, the increase of LPLA was not significant in the group (Figure 8). This finding indicates that the LPLA of skeletal muscle increases also in well-trained subjects when the physical work continues for very long periods of time and is very heavy. The mechanisms for this increase are unknown and are at present the subject of further investigations.

Acknowledgments

This work was supported by grants from the Swedish Medical Research Council (B80-19X-5446-02 and B80-19P-5640-01).

References

Brunzell, J., Chait, A., and Bierman, E.L. 1978. Pathophysiology of lipoprotein transport. *Metabolism* **27**:1109-1127.

Hermansen, L., Hultman, E., and Saltin, B. 1967. Muscle glycogen during prolonged severe exercise. *Acta Physiol. Scand.* **71**:129-139.

Linder, C., Chernick, S.S., Fleck, T.R., and Scow, R.O. 1976. Lipoprotein lipase and uptake of chylomicron triglyceride by skeletal muscle of rats. *Am. J. Physiol.* **231**:860-864.

Lithell, H., and Boberg, J. 1978. Determination of lipoprotein-lipase activity in human skeletal muscle tissue. *Biochim. Biophys. Acta* (Amsterdam) **528**:58-68.

Lithell, H., Boberg, J., Hellsing, K., Lundqvist, G., and Vessby, B. 1978. Lipoprotein-lipase activity in human skeletal muscle and adipose tissue in the fasting and the fed states. *Atherosclerosis* **30**:89-94.

Lithell, H., Hellsing, K., Lundqvist, G., and Malmberg, P. 1979. Lipoprotein-lipase activity of human skeletal muscle and adipose tissue after intensive physical exercise. *Acta Physiol. Scand.* **105**:312-315.

Lithell, H., Orlander, J., Schele, R., Sjodin, B., and Karlsson, J. 1979. Changes in lipoprotein-lipase activity and lipid stores in human skeletal muscle with prolonged heavy exercise. *Acta Physiol. Scand.* **107**:257-261.

Lithell, H., Cedermark, M., Fröberg, J., Tesch, P., and Karlsson, J. 1981. Increase of lipoprotein-lipase activity in skeletal muscle during heavy exercise. *Metabolism.* **30**:1130-1134.

Nikkilä, E., Torsti, P., and Penttila, P. 1963. The effect of exercise on lipoprotein lipase activity of rat heart, adipose tissue and skeletal muscle. *Metabolism* **12**:863-865.

Pykalisto, O. 1970. *Regulation of the Adipose-tissue Lipoprotein Lipase by Free Fatty Acids.* Thesis, University of Helsinki, Helsinki, Finland.

Rossner, S. 1974. Studies on an intravenous fat-tolerance test. Methodological, experimental, and clinical experiences with intralipid. *Acta Med. Scand., Suppl.* **564**.

Role of the Sympathetic Nervous System in Training-Induced Changes

Mikko Harri
University of Kuopio
Finland

Intense physical exercise is known to cause activation of the sympathoadrenal system. Prolonged activation of the sympathetic system occurs, for example, in exposure and acclimation to cold, and it has been shown that this activation is responsible for the many adaptive changes associated with cold acclimation (Harri and Valtola, 1975; Hsieh and Wang, 1971). Because many of the cold-induced changes, i.e., increased heart size, increased capacity for oxidative metabolism, and decreased heart rate (Harri and Valtola, 1975; Tirri et al., 1974) are similar to those caused by strenuous physical exercise, it is tempting to conclude that sympathetic activity bouts associated with the exercise periods may be necessary for an efficient adaptation to physical training.

Training Without Sympathetic Activation

The first method to elucidate the role of the sympathetic system for the training-induced changes is to modulate the level of sympathetic activity while keeping the amount of exercise constant. In these studies, the sympathetic influence was blocked by 6-hydroxydopamine (6-OH-DA), which causes a long-lasting degeneration of the adrenergic nerves (Sigvardsson et al., 1977) or by using beta-adrenergic blocking drugs, which block the influence of the released catecholamines at their receptor site (Harri and Narvola, 1979). An enlarged heart and a decreased heart rate at rest and at all work load levels are the known results of long-term physical training. Training also leads to an increase in cardiac receptor sensitivity to catecholamines (Wyatt et al., 1978), to increased tolerance to cold (Keatinge, 1961; Stromme and Hammel, 1967), and to certain

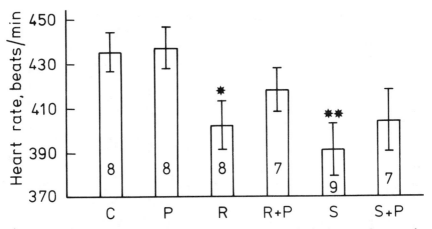

Figure 1—The resting heart rates in pentobarbital anesthetized rats. C—controls, P—propranolol-treated rats (10 mg/kg daily for 6 weeks), R—running-trained rats (1 hr. daily for 6 weeks), S—swimming-trained rats (3 hr. daily for 6 weeks). R + P and S + P indicate the rats which were injected with propranolol immediately before the daily running or swimming training. Vertical bars indicate ± SE. The numbers within the columns indicate the number of rats used. Asterisks indicate those values which were significantly different from the control: *$p < 0.05$ and **$p < 0.01$. From: Harri and Narvola, 1979.

metabolic adaptations in skeletal muscle metabolism (Vihko et al., 1978) to such an extent that these parameters are of importance in estimating physical fitness.

In rats trained after the 6-OH-DA injection (Sigvardsson et al., 1977) or under the influence of beta blockade (Harri and Narvola, 1979), however, the cardiac enlargement was smaller than in the rats trained without any drug treatment, despite an equal amount of exercise. Moreover, Figure 1 shows that in the animal groups trained under the influence of beta blockade no training bradycardia was observed. In addition, a reduction of the exercise heart rates at various work load levels can be obtained in normal rats but not in sympathectomized rats (Sigvardsson et al., 1977).

The results in Figure 2 show that trained rats have a greater response in the form of tachycardia to a beta-adrenergic drug, isoprenaline. Furthermore, the tachycardia in response to isoprenaline is smaller in the animal groups who performed their exercise sessions under the influence of beta blockade.

Figure 3 shows that trained rats maintained a higher skin temperature than did the controls at cold. Here again, in the animals having performed their training under the influence of beta blockade, the tail skin temperature stabilized at a lower level.

The results in Table 1 show that the responses of skeletal muscle variables to physical training are also dependent on sympathetic activa-

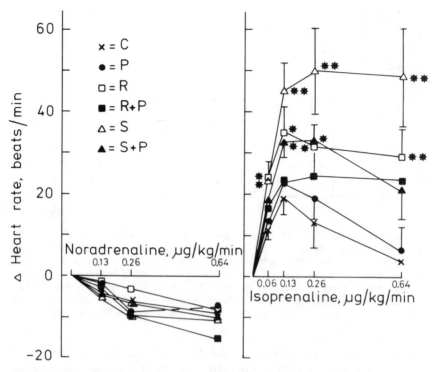

Figure 2—Effect of noradrenaline and isoprenaline infusions on heart rate in anesthetized rats. Responses that differ significantly from controls are marked by asterisks: *$p < 0.05$, **$p < 0.01$. Other explanations as in Figure 1. From: Harri and Narvola, 1979.

tion. This is demonstrated by the finding that beta blockade associated with training hampered the development of the enzymatic changes in skeletal muscle (unpublished data). That the amount of muscular work is not the only reason for the extent of enzymatic changes can be demonstrated by the swimming training in cool (30 °C) and warm waters (38 °C), respectively. In warm water, the rats swam very vigorously, whereas in cold water, they merely floated. Nevertheless, the enzymatic changes in skeletal muscle were as great or even greater in cold water swimmers than in warm water swimmers (unpublished data). The sympathetic activation is, of course, much higher in the former group because of threatening hypothermia.

Increased calorigenic sensitivity to injected noradrenaline is one of the manifestations of cold acclimation. Because repeated injections of exogenous noradrenaline can induce similar changes, the conclusion that increased sympathetic activity is the reason for this change is justified (Harri, 1978; Hsieh and Wang, 1971). Our results show, however, that swimming training but not running training resulted in increased

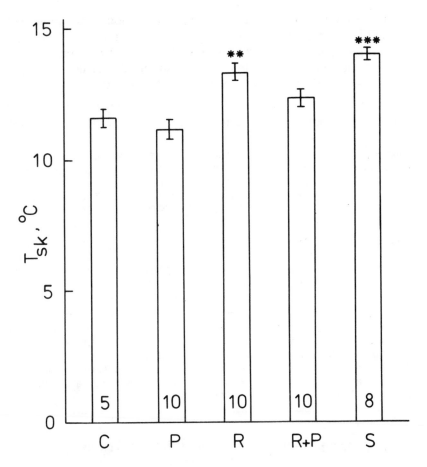

Figure 3—The stabilized tail skin temperature in rats exposed to 5 °C. Other explanations as in Figure 1. From: Harri, 1979.

calorigenic response to noradrenaline (Figure 4). This response was less marked in the animal group which had trained under the influence of beta blockade. Our further experiments have shown that the calorigenic sensitization is absent following swimming training in hyperthermic water temperature (38 °C), whereas the extent of sensitization is increased following training in cool water (30 °C) (unpublished data). This finding indicates that the greater thermoregulatory endurance of cold water swimming places more demands on the sympathetic system, which forms a major part of the thermoregulatory machinery, than does exercise alone. Furthermore, even very marked sympathetic activation during periods of running is—because of its short duration—not enough to sensitize the organism to the calorigenic action of noradrenaline.

Table 1—Effect of 6-week Running Training Without Propranolol (R)
and Under the Influence of 10 mg/kg of Propranolol (R + P)
on Skeletal Muscle Enzymes in M. Extensor Digit. Longus
(Typical Fast-Twitch Muscle) and in M. Soleus
(Typical Slow-Twitch Muscle) in Rats

Muscle	Enzyme	Controls	P	R	R + P
M. extensor	HADH	6.96	7.30	9.39[c]	9.26[b]
digit. longus	SDH	2.86	3.15	4.58[b]	3.93[a]
	CS	6.61	7.01	10.37[c]	10.10[c]
	MDH	118.00	119.00	147.00[b]	147.00[b]
	LDH	874.00	889.00	813.00	809.00[a]
M. soleus	HADH	21.9	22.1	27.6[c]	24.9
	SDH	4.47	4.96	5.86[b]	4.74
	CS	9.04	10.11	12.13[c]	11.36[b]
	MDH	211.00	221.00	259.00[c]	236.00[a]
	LDH	329.00	351.00	319.00	293.00

Note. P = rats treated by daily injections of propranolol only, HADH = 3-hydroxyacyl-CoA-dehydrogenase, CS = citrate synthase, SDH = succinate dehydrogenase, MDH = malate dehydrogenase, LDH = lactate dehydrogenase. Enzyme activities are expressed as moles of substrate utilized per min per g wet weight at 37 °C. Footnotes accompany those values which differ significantly from the controls: [a]$p<0.05$, [b]$p<0.01$, [c]$p<0.001$.

Sympathetic Activation Without Training

The results presented above demonstrate that blockade of the sympathetic influence during exercise periods greatly hampers the development of the training-induced adaptive changes. The second approach to the problem is to elucidate whether or not increased sympathetic activity per se can induce similar changes in the organism as does long-term physical training.

The results of experiments (Harri and Valtola, 1975) indeed show that cold-induced sympathetic activation as well as repeated stimulation of the adrenergic beta receptors by daily isoprenaline injections stimulate the activities of oxidative muscle enzymes in a way similar to swimming. On the other hand, severe heat, such as a sauna bath, also produces marked long-lasting activation of the sympathoadrenal system (Hussi et al., 1977). The experiments on rats show that even heat exposures, when repeated often enough, can activate the oxidative metabolism of the skeletal muscle (Harri, 1977).

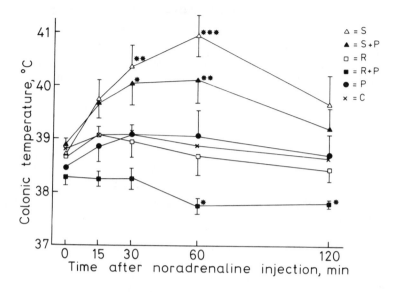

Figure 4—The response of the colonic temperature to injected noradrenaline (0.5 mg/kg i.p.) at 28 °C in rats. Other explanations as in Figure 1. From: Harri and Narvola, 1979.

Conclusions

The present results demonstrate that sympathetic blockade during the exercise periods hampers and an elevated sympathetic tone enhances the adaptive changes, commonly considered to be training dependent. They also show that prolonged sympathetic activation alone can induce very similar alterations in the same parameters as do standardized treadmill or swimming programs. These results support the conclusion that an adrenergic nervous system is necessary for an efficient adaptation to physical training.

This conclusion leads to many practical consequences. In more developed countries, for example, the number of aging persons using beta blockers or other sympatholytic drugs to control their diseases is increasing. It is also recommended that physical training should be included in their rehabilitation programs. As stated previously, the drug itself can very drastically alter the response to physical training. For this reason, training programs must be planned to fit individual demands, taking into account not only the disease but also the drugs used.

Acknowledgments

This research was supported by grants (8731/78/77 and 8224/78/78) from the Ministry of Education, Finland. Valuable technical assistance by Mr. Heikki Ronkko is greatly appreciated. Propranolol was a generous gift from the Imperial Chemical Industries (ICI, England).

References

Harri, M.N.E. 1977. Metabolic effects of repeated short-term exposures to heat in the rat. *Med. Biol.* **55**:330-333.

Harri, M.N.E. 1978. Metabolic and cardiovascular responses to prolonged noradrenaline load and their antagonism by beta blockade in the rat. *Acta Physiol. Scand.* **104**:402-414.

Harri, M.N.E. 1979. Physical training under the influence of beta blockade in rats. II. Effects on vascular reactivity. *Eur. J. Appl. Physiol.* **42**:151-157.

Harri, M.N.E. and Narvola, I. 1979. Physical training under the influence of beta blockade in rats: Effect on adrenergic responses. *Eur. J. Appl. Physiol.* **41**:199-210.

Harri, M.N.E., and Valtola, J. 1975. Comparison of the effects of physical exercise, cold acclimation, and repeated injections of isoprenaline on rat muscle enzymes. *Acta Physiol. Scand.* **95**:391-399.

Hsieh, A.C.L. and Wang, J.C.C. 1971. Colorigenic response to cold of rats after prolonged infusion of norepinephrine. *Am. J. Physiol.* **221**:335-337.

Hussi, E., Sonck, T., Poso, H., Remes, J., and Janne, J. 1977. Plasma catecholamines in Finnish sauna. *Ann. Clin. Res.* **9**:301-404.

Keatinge, W.R. 1961. The effect of repeated daily exposure to cold and of improved physical fitness on the metabolic and vascular response to cold air. *J. Physiol.*(London)**157**:209-220.

Sigvardsson, K., Sanfeldt, E., and Kilbom, A. 1977. Role of the adrenergic nervous system in development of training-induced bradycardia. *Acta Physiol. Scand.***101**:481-488.

Stromme, S.B. and Hammel, H.T. 1967. Effects of physical training on tolerance to cold in rats. *J. Appl. Physiol.* **23**:815-824.

Tirri, R., Harri, M.N.E., and Laitinen, L. 1974. Lowered chronotropic sensitivity of rat and frog hearts to sympathomimetic amines following cold acclimation. *Acta Physiol. Scand.* **90**:260-266.

Vihko, V., Soimajarvi, J., Karvinen, E., Rahkila, P., and Havu, M. 1978. Lipid metabolism during exercise I. Physiological and biochemical characterization of normal healthy male subjects in relation to their physical fitness. *Eur. J. Appl. Physiol.* **39**:209-218.

Wyatt, H.L., Chuck, L., Rabinowitz, B., Tyberg, J.V., and Parmley, W.W. 1978. Enhanced cardiac response to catecholamines in physically trained cats. *Am. J. Physiol.* **234**:H608-H613.

Anaerobic
Threshold

The Physiological Background of Onset of Blood Lactate Accumulation (OBLA)

Bertil Sjödin, Rickard Schéle, and **Jan Karlsson**
National Defense Research Institute
and Karolinska Hospital, Stockholm, Sweden

Dag Linnarsson
Karolinska Institute, Stockholm, Sweden

Richard Wallensten
Karolinska sjukhuset, Stockholm, Sweden

It is a well-established and recognized fact that accumulation of lactate in the contracting muscles and circulating blood is directly and/or indirectly related to physical fatigue. Short-term exercise performance is closely related to maximal values for lactate in muscle and blood (Karlsson, 1971) as well as to pH values in the same tissues (Sahlin, 1978). Recently, it was also determined that low muscle lactate values (submaximal) affect muscle performance capacity (Tesch et al., 1978b).

The appearance of lactate in muscle and blood has been suggested to be related to lack of molecular oxygen in the contracting muscles. A close relationship has been demonstrated between occurrence of lactate in contracting muscles and low oxygen saturation values in venous effluent from the contracting muscles (Jorfeldt et al., 1978; Saltin et al., 1971). It has been shown, however, that one of the two main muscle fiber types constituting skeletal muscle tissue in humans (fast twitch, FT, or type II fibers) has a marked glycogenolytic metabolic profile as compared with the other (slow twitch, ST, or type I fibers) (Sjödin, 1976). Thus, it seems reasonable to suggest that a specific recruitment of type II fibers might lead to excess lactate formation even if no true lack of molecular oxygen in the contracting muscles exists. Lactate formation might be related not only to the intensity of the exercise but also to the metabolic profile of the contracting muscle expressed as percentage of fast twitch or type II

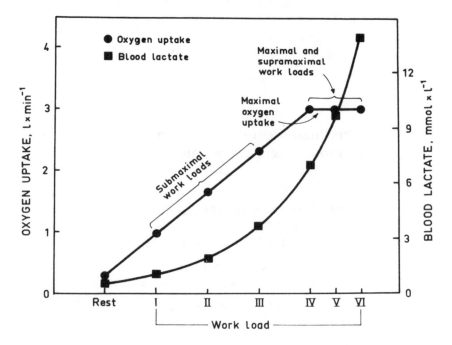

Figure 1—The "classical illustration" of the relationship between blood lactate concentration and exercise intensity under steady state or apparent steady state conditions.

fibers in the muscle.

It has been demonstrated that people who in their occupational work perform heavy exercise tend to work at an intensity not exceeding 50-60% of their maximal oxygen intake ($\dot{V}_{O_2}$ max) (Astrand and Rodahl, 1977), and it was pointed out that this relative work load coincided with the onset of blood lactate accumulation (Figure 1). It has been suggested that the relationship between lactate accumulation and fatigue may explain this preferred work intensity (for references, see Karlsson, 1971). These considerations have been the basis for including not only a measure of the cardiorespiratory fitness (e.g., maximal oxygen uptake) but also the blood lactate concentration at a submaximal work load to define athletes' exercise performance capacity.

A modification of this testing approach has recently been developed and the exercise intensity or the oxygen uptake corresponding to a certain submaximal lactate concentration has been used to predict exercise performance capacity. Because muscle and blood lactate, in addition to pH, will affect respiration, it has been suggested that changes in respiratory variables such as the relationship between respiratory exchange ratio (R) and oxygen uptake can be used similarly for determination of the "lactate breaking point" and/or the "anaerobic threshold" (MacDougall,

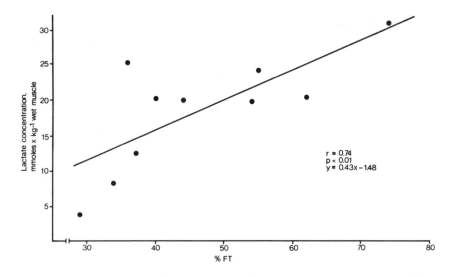

Figure 2—The relationship between muscle lactate concentration and percentage of fast twitch (percentage of FT) fibers in the vastus lateralis muscle after short-term maximal exercise (Tesch et al., 1978a).

1977; Mader et al., 1976; and Wasserman et al., 1964). The validity of these expressions is somewhat doubtful, inasmuch as the cause of the appearance of lactate in human skeletal muscle during exercise is still obscure. It has already been pointed out that the reason might be a true lack of oxygen; but it is also possible that an excess lactate formation only, or predominantly, in the fast twitch motor units can affect mixed muscle tissue or blood lactate concentrations. (Tesch, 1980).

Lactate accumulation in the muscle during short-term (5-10 min.) exercise depends upon muscle fiber composition expressed as a percentage of fast twitch fibers (Karlsson, 1980) (Figure 2). It is also possible to demonstrate that lactate accumulation will increase more with a larger calculated oxygen deficit at the onset of exercise (Karlsson, 1971) (Figure 3). In this experimental situation, lactate formation is related to the fact that the ATP synthesizing processes are in a transient condition, i.e., no metabolic steady state has been established (Linnarsson, 1974). The muscle and blood lactate concentration values obtained within 10 min. of onset of exercise is to a large extent affected by a steady state not being established immediately at the onset of exercise. The relevancy of the common practice of relating blood lactate concentration in a transient condition to oxygen uptake at steady state, as in Figure 1, can thus be questioned.

By means of frequent lactate concentration determinations in arterial

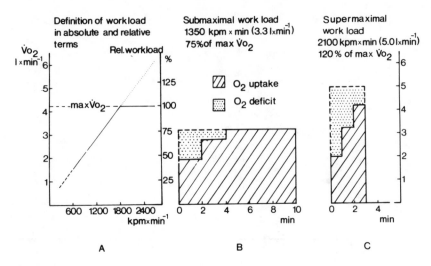

Figure 3a—Calculation of oxygen deficit at submaximal and maximal bicycle exercise (Karlsson, 1971).

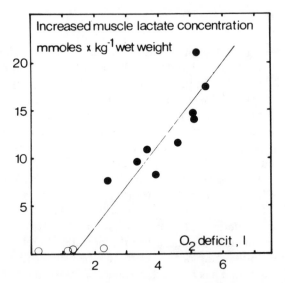

Figure 3b—The relationship between the increase in lactate concentration and oxygen deficit at submaximal and maximal bicycle exercise (Karlsson, 1971).

and venous blood over exercising muscles at different work loads and after approximately 15 min. of exercise, it is possible to establish the exercise intensity whenever an onset of blood lactate accumulation is expressed as a positive venous-arterial lactate difference (Jorfeldt et al.,

Arterial concentrations and fv – a diff for lactate ● and pyruvate

mmoles × l^{-1}

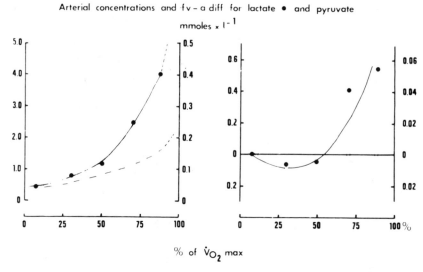

Figure 4—Arterial pyruvate and lactate concentration and venous-arterial concentration differences over the exercising leg (data from Jorfeldt et al., 1978).

1978) (Figure 4). Based on similar experimental protocols, it is possible to demonstrate that an Onset of Blood Lactate Accumulation (OBLA) in the body exists, expressed as a release of lactate from the exercising muscles at work loads in excess of 60-70% of maximal oxygen uptake (Figure 5). These data have been obtained under conditions which were assumed to be close to or possibly identical with "true" steady state conditions in the contracting muscles. A similar experimental protocol is exercise with stepwise increases in intensity, starting with, for example, loadless pedaling or walking (Linnarsson, 1974). Oxygen deficit periods will thus be markedly reduced and the lactate concentration determined in the blood is more a mirror of the metabolic state in the contracting muscles as described, rather than a reflection of transient metabolic stages. Such protocols are the basis for the OBLA test in our laboratory (Figure 6), the lactate breaking point test, and for the anaerobic threshold test by Mader and Wasserman and their collaborators. These protocols have, in a number of studies, been applied to bicycle exercise as well as treadmill running.

One may question to what extent tests, such as the OBLA test, are complimentary to determination of individual maximal oxygen uptake or can act as a substitute for this classical measure of physical capacity. The capacity for prolonged running (5,000 m) expressed as average speed during the race showed correlations with maximal oxygen uptake in the order of .60 to .80 (Figure 7), which is in agreement with a number of

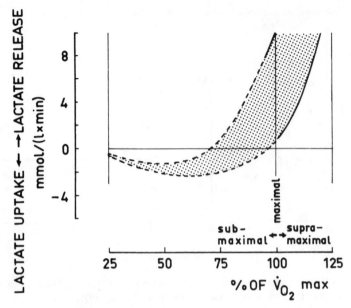

Figure 5—Estimation of lactate metabolism over the leg during standarized bicycle exercise during steady state conditions (Karlsson, 1980).

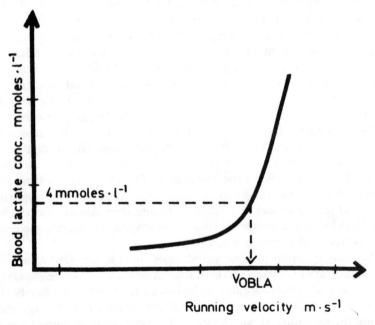

Figure 6—Definition of running speed corresponding to a blood lactate concentration of 4 mmoles $\times$ 1^{-1}. This concentration is referred to as the value corresponding to OBLA.

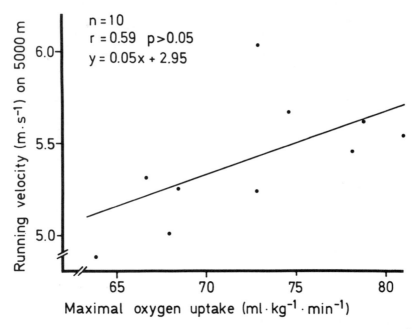

Figure 7—Mean running velocity at 5,000 m in relation to maximal oxygen uptake ($\dot{V}_{O_2}$ max, ml $\times$ kg^{-1} x min^{-1}).

previous studies (for references, see Davies and Thompson, 1979). When the performance capacity in the races was related to the speed which corresponds to OBLA (V_{OBLA}) a correlation coefficient in the order of .90 was obtained (Figure 8). This means that in the examined samples (i.e., subjects used to regular training, though not at elite levels) better predictions were obtained by using the OBLA test than by using maximal oxygen intake. In addition, it is worth emphasizing that an interrelationship has been established between V_{OBLA} and biomechanical features of endurance running (Komi et al., 1981).

What then is the physiological background for these relationships and the higher predictability of the OBLA test? One way to approach this question is to examine individual differences at submaximal exercise intensities and then to relate them to the OBLA test results. When this was done, it was found that subjects with a higher oxygen uptake at a given submaximal running speed (i.e., subjects with a low running economy) also had a lower speed corresponding to OBLA (Figure 9). When the oxygen uptake was expressed in percent of maximal oxygen uptake, an even higher correlation with V_{OBLA} was obtained (Figure 10). Subjects with a high OBLA utilized a lower fraction of their maximal oxygen uptake at the given submaximal running speed. In conclusion, onset of lactate ac-

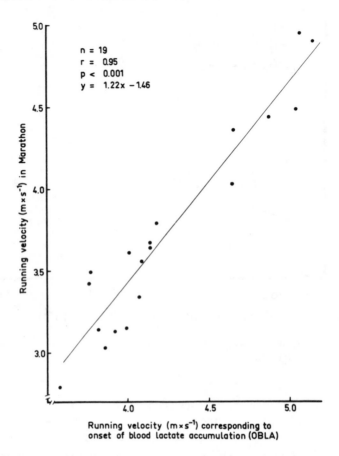

Figure 8—Mean running velocity during a marathon race and running velocity corresponding to OBLA (V_{OBLA}) (see Figure 7).

cumulation in muscle and blood at low speeds occurs in conjunction with a poor running economy. It is tempting to explain this finding using the data reported by Tesch and collaborators (Tesch, 1978, 1980; Tesch et al., 1978a, 1978b), which suggests that muscle contractility is impaired due to local lactate accumulation. An early onset of lactate accumulation or a higher level of lactate accumulation are in a number of exercise situations related to a higher percentage of FT muscle fibers in the contracting muscles (Tesch et al., 1978a). In running, this can be illustrated by the positive correlation between V_{OBLA} and the percentage of slow twitch fibers (Figure 11). The percentage of maximal oxygen uptake corresponding to the blood lactate concentration of 4 mmoles $\times 1^{-1}$ was also positively related to percentage of slow twitch fibers (Figure 12).

It is well established that endurance training improves cardio-

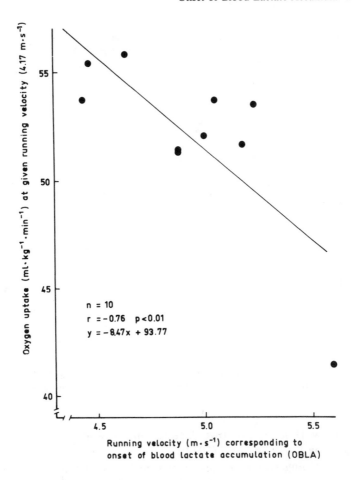

Figure 9—Running velocity at a submaximal speed (4.7 m $\times$ s^{-1} or 17 km $\times$ h^{-1}) and running velocity corresponding to OBLA (V$_{OBLA}$) .

respiratory functions and that the increased maximal oxygen uptake is usually considered a consequence thereof. Recently, it was demonstrated that local changes in muscle fiber composition can also occur (Jansson et al., 1978): the percentage of FTb fibers may decrease, whereas the percentage of FTa and the percentage of ST fibers increase indicating a transformation of FTb via FTa to ST fibers. The FTb fiber is the most glycogenolytic and most fatiguable (for references, see Tesch, 1980). Indications are also present that endurance training will shift the LDH isozyme patterns in both fiber types to a higher proportion of the heart muscle specific LDH isozyme (LDH-1) (Sjodin, 1976). This might decrease the rate of lactate production and accumulation in the fibers at

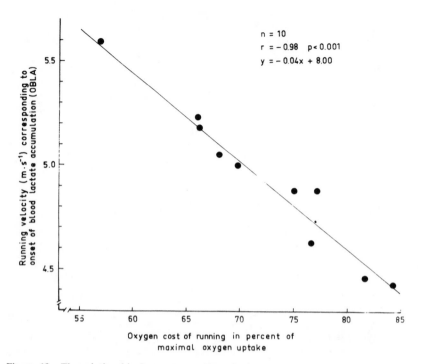

Figure 10—The relationship between running velocity corresponding to OBLA (V_{OBLA}) and the oxygen uptake at 4.7 m × s⁻¹ in percentage of maximal oxygen uptake.

submaximal work loads and lower lactate concentration will be obtained as indicated by Karlsson et al. (1972).

In most training studies it has been possible to demonstrate an increased maximal oxygen uptake (Grimby and Saltin, 1971). Studies in which the kinetics of lactate production are studied simultaneously with oxygen uptake have been rare. Some of them have either failed to demonstrate increases or shown only small increases in maximal oxygen uptake but demonstrated increases in relative exercise loads corresponding to onset of blood lactate accumulation (Karlsson et al., 1972), i.e., after training $\dot{V}_{O_2}$ max. might change in terms of OBLA as speculated in by MacDougall (1977) or in a corresponding measure.

Because endurance capacity is one of the most prominent features in the concept of physical performance capacity, a number of methods have been developed to test this trait. Most of the tests have been based on measurements for cardiorespiratory variables such as oxygen uptake, respiratory rate, and heart rate at submaximal and maximal levels. Heart rate data obtained at submaximal exercise levels have often been extrapolated to estimate maximal values for oxygen uptake. Other test pro-

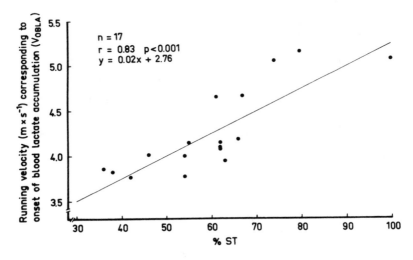

Figure 11—The relationship between running velocity corresponding to OBLA (V_{OBLA}) and muscle fiber composition in the vastus lateralis muscle.

cedures have had a more practical design in which the amount of work performed under some specified conditions usually leading to exhaustion, such as time for a certain distance or distances covered during a specified time, has been used as an expression of physical performance capacity. With the exception of determination of maximal oxygen uptake and maximal tests where the amount of work has been defined, these methods have low precision and low validity as measures of the individual exercise performance capacity.

Because endurance capacity is one of the most prominent features in the concept of physical performance capacity, a number of methods have been developed to test for this trait. Most of the tests have been based on measurements for cardiorespiratory variables such as oxygen uptake, respiratory R, and heart rate at submaximal and maximal levels. Heart rate data obtained at submaximal exercise levels have often been extrapolated to estimate maximal values for oxygen uptake. Other test procedures have had a more practical design in which the amount of work performed under some specified conditions usually leading to exhaustion, such as time for a certain distance or distances covered during a specified time, has been used as an expression of physical performance capacity. With the exception of determination of maximal oxygen uptake and maximal tests where the amount of work has been defined, these methods have low precision and low validity as measures of the individual exercise performance capacity.

A submaximal exercise test is to be preferred to a maximal (exhaustive)

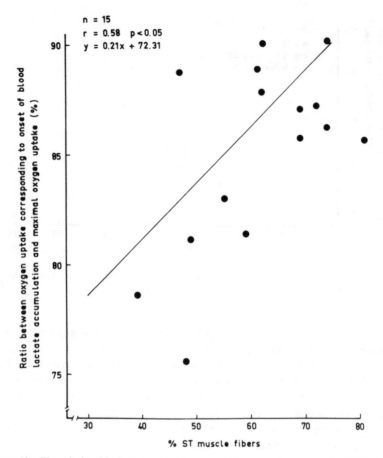

Figure 12—The relationship between oxygen uptake corresponding to onset of OBLA expressed as percentage of maximal oxygen uptake and muscle fiber composition in the vastus lateralis muscle.

test when the risk for complications cannot be determined in advance. A submaximal testing procedure is also preferable in prolonged exercise experiments, such as training sojourns and repeated testing during daily occupational work. The OBLA test and similar procedures are true submaximal tests. An experienced investigator will interrupt the experiments or the tests at exercise intensities which are far from maximal. Because this test procedure has been proven to be superior to determinations of maximal oxygen uptake in many situations and conditions, for example, testing of top athletes and evaluation of their performance capacity, it seems reasonable to suggest that the OBLA test would be a satisfactory test to apply in many other situations. For athletes, it seems reasonable to suggest determinations of maximal oxygen uptake and OBLA. The relationship between oxygen uptake corresponding to OBLA and the maximal oxygen uptake could be a measure of the efficiency of the endurance training. A large difference would indicate an inefficient endurance program, whereas a smaller difference could indicate that more emphasis could be spent on training programs to improve maximal oxygen uptake. The OBLA test can be performed as treadmill exercise as well as bicycle exercise. Thus, the OBLA test during bicycle exercise could be a satisfactory field method to assess exercise performance capacity.

Acknowledgment

This study was supported by grants from the Swedish Medical Research Council (Project No.4251) and the Research Council of the Swedish Sports Federation.

References

Astrand, P.-O., and Rodahl, K. 1977. *Textbook of Work Physiology.* McGraw-Hill Book Co.,New York, NY.

Davies, C.T.M., and Thompson, M.W. 1979. Aerobic performance of female marathon and male ultramarathon athletes. *Eur. J. Appl. Physiol.* 41:233-245.

Grimby, G., and Saltin, B. 1971. Physiological effects of physical training. *Scand. J. Rehab. Med.* 3:31-38.

Jansson, E., Sjodin, B., and Tesch, P. 1978. Changes in muscle fibre type distribution in man after physical training. *Acta Physiol. Scand.* 104:235-237.

Jorfeldt, L., Juhlin-Dannfelt, A., and Karlsson, J. 1978. Lactate release in relation to tissue lactate in human skeletal muscle during exercise. *J. Appl. Physiol.: Respirat. Environ. Exercise Physiol.* 44(3):350-352.

Karlsson, J. 1971. Lactate and phosphagen concentrations in working muscle of man (with special reference to oxygen deficit at the onset of work). *Acta Physiol Scand.;* Suppl. 358.

Karlsson, J. 1980. Localized muscular fatigue: Role of muscle metabolism and substrate depletion. In: R.S. Hutton (ed.). *Exercise and Sport Sciences Reviews.* Franklin Institute Press, Philadelphia, PA.

Karlsson, J., Nordesjo, L.-O., and Saltin, B. 1972. Muscle lactate, ATP, and CP levels during exercise after physical training in man. *J. Appl. Physiol.* 33:199-203.

Komi, P.V., Ito, A., Sjodin, B., and Karlsson, J. 1981. Muscle metabolism, lactate breaking point and biomechanical features of endurance running. *Int. J. Sports Med.* 2:148-153.

Linnarsson, D. 1974. Dynamics of pulmonary gas exchange and heart rate changes at start and end of exercise. *Acta Physiol. Scand.,* Suppl. 415.

MacDougall, J.D. 1977. The anaerobic threshold: its significance for the endurance athlete. *Can. J. Appl. Sport Sci.* **2**:137-140.

Mader, A., Liesen, H., Hech, H., Phillippi, H., Rost, R., Schurch, P., and Hollman, W. 1976. Zur Beurteilung der Sportart Spezifischen Ausdauer-leistungsfahigkeit in Labor. *Sportarzt und Sportmed.* **4**:80-84.

Sahlin, K. 1978. Intracellular pH and energy metaboism in skeletal muscle of man (with special reference to exercise). *Acta Physiol. Scand.,* Suppl. **455**.

Saltin, B., Gollnick, P.D., Piehl, K., and Eriksson, B. 1971. Metabolic and cir-culatory adjustments at onset of exercise. In: A. Gilbert and P. Guille (eds.) *Onset of Exercise,* pp.63-76. University of Toulouse, Toulouse, France.

Sjodin, B. 1976. Lactate dehydrogenase in human skeletal muscle. *Acta Physiol. Scand.,* Suppl. **436**.

Tesch, P. 1978. Local lactate and exhaustion. *Acta Physiol Scand.* **104**:373-374.

Tesch, P. 1980. Fatigue pattern in subtypes of human skeletal muscle fibers. *Int. J. Sports Med.* **1**:79-81.

Tesch, P., Sjodin, B., and Karlsson, J. 1978a. Relationship between lactate ac-cumulation, LDH activity, LDH isozyme, and fiber type distribution in human skeletal muscle. *Acta Physiol. Scand.* **103**:40-46.

Tesch, P., Sjodin., B., Thorstensson, A., and Karlsson, J. 1978b. Muscle fatigue and its relation to lactate accumulation and LDH activity in man. *Acta Physiol. Scand.* **103**:413-420.

Wasserman, K., and McIlroy, M.B. 1964. Detecting the threshold of anaerobic metabolism in cardiac patients during exercise. *Am. J. Cardiol.* **14**:844-852.

The Relationships Among Running Economy, Aerobic Power, Muscle Power, and Onset of Blood Lactate Accumulation in Young Boys (11-15 Years)

Bertil Sjödin
National Defense Research Institute
and Karolinska Hospital, Stockholm, Sweden

In several investigations, different physiological factors have been studied in relation to running performance. Most studies are cross-sectional and deal with adults, whereas the present investigation, ongoing for 2 years, is a longitudinal study of young boys. Sixteen boys, 11-15 years old, from two athletic clubs, have participated in the study. The boys are middle and long distance runners. Thus, the emphasis in their training has been endurance oriented, but some specific strength and sprint training have also been included.

The boys and their parents have given their informed consent to participate in the study.

Methods

The following test protocol is performed twice a year: Aerobic power (i.e., maximal oxygen uptake) is determined during uphill running on a treadmill using the Douglas bag method.

Muscle power is measured with a strength endurance test according to Thorstensson (1976). This is performed as a one-leg exercise of 100 repeated maximal knee extensions at an angular velocity of 300° per second on an isokinetic dynamometer (Cybex II). The peak torque generated during each of the first 50 knee extensions is cumulated and used as an index of muscle power.

The running velocity corresponding to the onset of blood lactate ac-

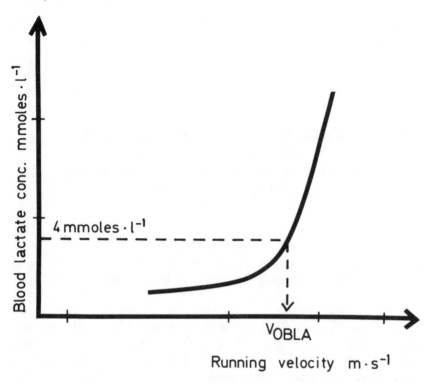

Figure 1—Blood lactate concentration in relation to running velocity. The velocity corresponding to a blood lactate concentration of 4 mmoles $\times$ 1^{-1} is defined as the velocity corresponding to onset of blood lactate accumulation (V_{OBLA}).

cumulation (V_{OBLA}) is determined during submaximal running on a treadmill. The velocity is increased every fourth minute. Blood samples for lactate concentration determinations are taken during the last minute at each velocity. V_{OBLA} is defined as the velocity corresponding to a blood lactate concentration of 4 mmoles $\times$ -6' (Figure 1). Oxygen uptake is determined simultaneously at each velocity. Oxygen uptake (ml $\times$ kg^{-1} $\times$ min^{-1}) at a given velocity (17 km $\times$ h^{-1}) is used as an index of running economy ($\dot{V}_{O_2}17$).

Results and Discussion

The subjects have been tested with the complete protocol on four occasions. The observation period included two competition seasons, 1977 and 1978. During this period, maximal oxygen uptake and muscle power expressed in absolute terms increased significantly. The increase in maximal oxygen uptake was related to the increase in body weight over the

Table 1—Changes in Maximal Oxygen Uptake ($\dot{V}_{O_2}$ max) and
Muscular Power ($\pm SD$) Between 1977 and 1978 in Young Boys

	$\dot{V}_{O_2}$ max		Muscular power	
	$l \times min^{-1}$	$ml \times kg^{-1} \times min^{-1}$	Nm	$Nm \times kg^{-1}$
1977	2.3 ± 0.3	65.0 ± 3.2	1790 ± 412	50.3 ± 7.7
1978	2.5 ± 0.3	65.7 ± 3.2	2240 ± 532	57.1 ± 7.1
p	0.001	n.s.	0.001	0.05

Note. $n = 11$

period (Table 1).

On the first occasion the V_{OBLA} correlated highly with running economy ($r = -0.86$, $p < 0.001$) but not with aerobic power (n.s.); however, on later test occasions increasing relationships between V_{OBLA} and aerobic power ($r = 0.71$, $p = < 0.01$) were found, whereas the relationships to running economy decreased ($r = -0.53$, $p < 0.05$).

Thus, the velocity at which onset of blood lactate accumulation occurs seems to be dependent on at least two different factors: the aerobic power and the running economy. The onset of blood lactate accumulation may in some way reflect the optimal limit for the aerobic energy production system in the muscle tissue during exercise. This may explain the correlation with aerobic capacity. An intracellular accumulation of lactate also inhibits the muscle function and thus impairs the running economy. This may explain the correlation with running economy.

Maximal oxygen uptake, muscle power, and V_{OBLA} were also correlated with the subjects' highest running velocity for different running distances during one competitive season (Table 2). The velocities for 400, 1,000 and 3,000 m track running were highly correlated with the individual V_{OBLA}. Weaker relationships were present between the velocity for 400 and 1,000 m and the anaerobic capacity. Only the velocity for 4.2 km cross-country running was related to the aerobic capacity.

The velocity for 1,000 m track running showed a nonsignificant correlation to aerobic power ($r = 0.44$, $p > 0.05$) and a weak correlation with running economy, i.e., $\dot{V}_{O_2}$ at 17 km $\times$ h^{-1} ($r = -0.56$, $p < 0.05$). Note that the coefficient for $\dot{V}_{O_2}$ 17 is negative. Thus a *low* $\dot{V}_{O_2}$ 17 indicates *high* running economy.

The multiple correlation between velocity on 1,000 m track running, aerobic power and running economy was 0.85. The multiple regression equation generated was:

$$V_{1000} = 5.09 - 0.06 \, \dot{V}_{O_2} \, 17 + 0.06 \, \dot{V}_{O_2} \, max,$$

Table 2—Relationships Among Running Velocity During Different
Competition Distances, Maximal Oxygen Uptake ($\dot{V}_{O_2}$ max),
Muscular Power, and V_{OBLA} in Young Boys

Physiological factors		100 m $n = 11$	400 m $n = 9$	1,000 m $n = 14$	3,000 m $n = 11$	Cross-country running, 4.2 km $n = 8$
$\dot{V}_{O_2}$ max	r	0.35	0.51	0.47	0.48	0.77[a]
Muscular power	r	0.55	0.67[a]	0.59[a]	0.42	0.28
V_{OBLA}	r	0.50	0.86[b]	0.90[c]	0.89[c]	0.71

Note. [a]$p < 0.05$; [b]$p < 0.01$; [c]$p < 0.001$

where both $\dot{V}_{O_2}$ 17 and V_{O_2} max were significant factors ($p < 0.001$ and
$p < 0.01$). This indicates that a subject with relatively low aerobic capacity might compensate for this with a high running economy and vice versa. It should be emphasized that the subjects of this investigation were children. It is possible that the present results might be applicable to adults as well.

Acknowledgments

This study was supported by grants from the Swedish Medical Research Council (No. 4251) and the Research Council of the Swedish Sports Federation.

Reference

Thorstensson, A. 1976. Muscle strength, fibre types and enzyme activities in man. *Acta Physiol Scand,* Suppl. **443**.

Oxygen Cost of Treadmill Running
in Long Distance Runners

Bertil Sjödin and **Rickard Schéle**
National Defense Research Institute
and Karolinska Hospital, Stockholm, Sweden

It is well established that one of the typical features of the long distance runner is a high maximal oxygen uptake (Astrand and Rodahl, 1978; Saltin and Astrand, 1967). It is also known that, at a given submaximal exercise intensity, the energy expenditure per unit body weight will differ among runners (Costill and Fox, 1968). These individual differences can be the result of differences in equipment (e.g., footwear, as demonstrated by Turrell and Robinsson, 1943). If the energy cost during submaximal running is normalized for differences in body weight and clothing, for example, individual variation still exists (Costill and Fox, 1968), which might be due to a variation in mechanical efficiency. Individual variations in metabolic efficiency may also be an additional explanation. Recent studies have indicated that muscle fiber composition is of significance for the onset of blood lactate accumulation during submaximal running (Sjödin et al., 1982; Sjödin and Jacobs, 1981).

In order to further elucidate differences in energy expenditure, 10 experienced long distance runners have been studied with regard to running economy and some related physiological features.

Subjects and Methods

Ten experienced long distance runners were employed in the present study. They have participated in a number of studies and are well acquainted with the exercise test. The test consists of treadmill running with stepwise increasing velocity. Fingertip blood and oxygen uptake were obtained during the last (fourth) minute of each exercise load, i.e.,

Table 1—Some Characteristics of the 10 Subjects

Group characteristics	$\bar{x}$	Range
Age (years)	21	18-29
Weight (kg)	63.1	48.2-72.1
$\dot{V}_{O_2}$ max (ml $\times$ kg^{-1} $\times$ min^{-1})	72.5	63.8-81.0

during steady state conditions. Oxygen uptake was assessed by means of Douglas bag procedures and the expired gas was analyzed using a mass spectrometer (MGA 200, Centronics, London). Blood lactate was determined according to Strom (1949). Maximal oxygen uptake was determined during uphill running (3-5°) leading to exhaustion in 5-10 min. after the onset of running. The different physiological characteristics related to Onset of Blood Lactate Accumulation (OBLA) were obtained as presented by Sjodin et al. (1982).

Results

Mean values of age, weight, and maximal oxygen uptake ($\dot{V}_{O_2}$max) are given in Table 1. Oxygen uptake values at four submaximal running intensities were obtained for each individual and the relationship between oxygen uptake and running velocity was in all cases very high ($r > 0.99$). When all the individual data for oxygen uptake during submaximal running were pooled, a lower correlation was obtained ($r = 0.87$, $p < 0.001$) than that presented by Costill and Fox (1968) ($r = 0.95$). This indicated that the interindividual variation in oxygen cost of running was larger in the present study. The range of individual oxygen uptake at the same submaximal speed (15 km $\times$ h^{-1}) was wide ($\dot{V}_{O_2}$15:41.4-55.8 ml $\times$ kg^{-1} $\times$ min^{-1}). Running velocity corresponding to the onset of blood lactate accumulation (V_{OBLA}) also displayed great individual variations (4.41-5.57 m $\times$ s^{-1}). The runners also demonstrated large variations in competitive performances expressed as the mean velocity during 5,000 m track running ($V_{5,000} = 4.80$-6.03 m $\times$ s^{-1}). The correlation coefficients between the different physiological characteristics and performance are presented in Table 2. The oxygen cost of running at a velocity of 15 km $\times$ h^{-1} correlated best with V_{OBLA} ($r = -.76$): i.e., the higher the runner's speed at a blood lactate concentration of 4 mmol/1, the lower the oxygen uptake when running with a speed of 15 km $\times$ h^{-1}. The relative oxygen cost of running at a speed of 15 km $\times$ h^{-1}($\dot{V}_{O_2}$15/$\dot{V}_{O_2}$max) showed a very high negative correlation with V_{OBLA} ($r = -.98$). The

Table 2—Correlations Between Running Performance
and Physiological Measurements Obtained During Treadmill Exercise

	$\dot{V}_{O_2}$ 15 ml × kg^{-1} × min^{-1}	$\dfrac{\dot{V}_{O_2}\,15}{\dot{V}_{O_2}\,max}$ %	V_{OBLA} m × s^{-1}	$\dot{V}_{O_2}$ max ml × kg^{-1} × min^{-1}	V_{5000} m × s^{-1}
$\dot{V}_{O_2}$ 15 ml × kg^{-1} × min^{-1}			$-.76^a$	$-.02$	$-.74^a$
$\dfrac{\dot{V}_{O_2}\,15}{\dot{V}_{O_2}\,max}$ %			$-.98^c$		$-.94^c$
V_{OBLA} m × s^{-1}	$-.76^a$	$-.98^c$		$.65^a$	$.94^c$
$\dot{V}_{O_2}$ max ml × kg^{-1} × min^{-1}	$-.02$		$.65^a$		$.59$
V_{5000} m × s^{-1}	$-.74^a$	$-.94^c$	$.94^c$	$.59$	

Note. $n = 10$
[a] $p < 0.05$
[b] $p < 0.01$
[c] $p < 0.001$

64   Sjödin and Schéle

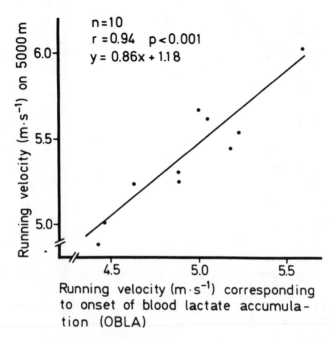

Figure 1a—The relationship between running velocity (m × s⁻¹) during 5,000 m and running velocity corresponding to onset of blood lactate accumulation (V_OBLA).

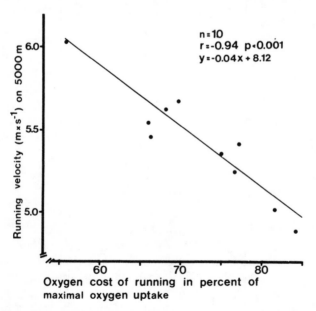

Figure 1b—The relationship between running velocity (m × s⁻¹) during 5,000 m and the relative oxygen cost of running (V̇_O,15/V̇_O,max).

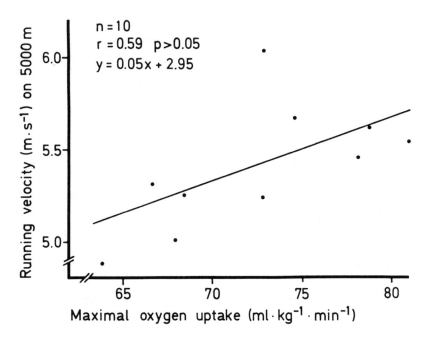

Figure 2—The relationship between running velocity (m × s⁻¹) during 5,000 m and maximal oxygen uptake ($\dot{V}_{O_2}$max, ml × kg⁻¹ × min⁻¹).

relative oxygen cost of running ($\dot{V}_{O_2}15/\dot{V}_{O_2}$max) and V_{OBLA} were both better correlated to $V_{5,000}$ (Figures 1a, 1b) than the classical measure of endurance capacity ($\dot{V}_{O_2}$ max) (Figure 2).

Multiple regression analysis indicated that both the oxygen cost of running at 15 km × h⁻¹ and $\dot{V}_{O_2}$ max are significant determinants of $V_{OBLA}(R = .98)$ and $V_{5,000}(R = .93)$. (Table 3). The multiple correlation coefficients were practically identical with the simple correlations obtained with the fraction $\dot{V}_{O_2}15/\dot{V}_{O_2}$ max ($r = -.98$ and $-.94$, respectively).

Discussion

The major finding in the present study was the large individual variation in oxygen uptake at a given submaximal running speed in spite of minimal variatiion in the weight of footwear and clothing. The variation was considerably greater than previously observed for long distance runners (Costill and Fox, 1968). It seems reasonable to suggest that the observed variation in the oxygen cost of running is mainly due to individual differences in running economy. The relative oxygen cost of

Table 3—Running Economy ($\dot{V}_{O_2}$ 15) and Maximal Oxygen Uptake ($\dot{V}_{O_2}$ max) as Determinants of Running Speed at Onset of Blood Lactate Accumulation (V_{OBLA}) and Speed in a 5,000 m Track Run (V_{5000}) [Regression equations, multiple regression coefficient (R) and standard deviation from regression (S_e)]

Multiple regression equation	R	S_e
V_{OBLA} = 8.42-0.067 $\dot{V}_{O_2}$ 15[a]	0.761	0.245
V_{OBLA} = 5.56-0.066 $\dot{V}_{O_2}$ 15[c] + 0.04 $\dot{V}_{O_2}$ max[c]	0.982	0.075
V_{5000} = 8.55-0.60 $\dot{V}_{O_2}$ 15[a]	0.736	0.234
V_{5000} = 6.09-0.059 $\dot{V}_{O_2}$ 15[b] + 0.033 $\dot{V}_{O_2}$ max[b]	0.933	0.136

Note. n = 10
[a]$p < 0.05$
[b]$p < 0.01$
[c]$p < 0.001$

running showed closer correlation to running performance ($V_{5,000}$) than did oxygen cost or maximal oxygen uptake when considered separately.

In earlier studies, it was possible to demonstrate a positive relationship between lactate accumulation and a high percentage of fast twitch muscle fibers in the exercising muscles (Tesch, 1980). A study of marathon runners also demonstrated that muscle fiber composition partly determines the onset of blood lactate accumulation during running (Sjödin and Jacobs, 1981). The causal relationship between an early onset of lactate accumulation in blood and low running economy is at present unclear and can only be speculated upon. It is possible that an increased local lactate accumulation affects muscle performance characteristics and subsequently increases the energy expenditure per unit of power output. It is also possible that a high oxygen uptake at a certain submaximal exercise load (i.e., a low running economy) is indicative of low mechanical efficiency of the running movement, which might increase the oxygen demand in the active muscles and subsequently cause an increased lactate formation and accumulation in the blood.

In summary, experienced runners demonstrated individual variations in oxygen uptake at a submaximal running speed, which were suggested to be the result of individual variations in running economy. The oxygen uptake when running at a speed of 15 km $\times$ h^{-1} was more highly related to lactate metabolism than to the individual capacity for oxygen uptake (maximal oxygen uptake). Both the differences in mechanical efficiency and/or in metabolic efficiency might cause the observed variations.

Acknowledgments

This study was supported by grants from the Swedish Medical Research Council (No.4251) and the Research Council of the Swedish Sports Federation.

References

Astrand, P-O., and Rodahl, K. 1977. *Textbook of Work Physiology.* McGraw-Hill Book Co., New York, NY.

Costill, D.L., and Fox, E.L. 1969. Energetics of marathon running. *Med. Sci. Sports* 1:81-86.

Saltin, B., and Astrand, P-O. 1967. Maximal oxygen uptake in athletics. *J. Appl. Physiol.* 23(3):353-358.

Sjödin, B., and Jacobs, I. 1981. Onset of blood lactate accumulation and marathon running performance. *Int. J. Sports Med.* 2:23-26.

Sjödin, B., Linnarsson, D., Wallensten, R., Schele, R., and Karlsson, J. 1982. The physiological background of onset of blood lactate accumulation (OBLA). In: P. Komi (ed.), *Exercise and Sport Biology*, Human Kinetics Publishers, Champaign, IL.

Strom, G. 1949. The influence of anoxia on lactate utilization in man after prolonged muscular work. *Acta Physiol. Scand.* 17:440-451.

Tesch, P. 1980. Muscle fatigue in man: With special reference to lactate accumulation during short-term intense exercise. *Acta Physiol. Scand., Suppl.* 480.

Turell, E.S., and Robinson, S. 1943. Interim Report No.3. Committee on Medical Research of the Office of Scientific Research and Development. December 31.

Maximum Oxygen Uptake, Anaerobic Threshold, and Skeletal Muscle Enzymes in Male Athletes

Heikki Rusko and **Paavo Rahkila**
University of Jyväskylä, Finland

During the past few years, the endurance of athletes has been physiologically characterized by measuring their anaerobic threshold, which might be a better measure than maximum oxygen uptake for evaluating the submaximal fitness and the performance capacity of endurance athletes (Mader et al., 1976; Weltman et al., 1978). Experiments on animals and on human subjects, including athletes, have shown that endurance training increases the oxidative capacity of muscles, which might be one of the most important determinants of prolonged endurance performance (Gollnick et al., 1972; Holloszy, 1967). In previous studies, statistically significant correlations between maximum oxygen uptake, oxidative enzyme activities, and muscle fiber composition have been observed (Bergh et al., 1978; Rusko et al., 1978). The purposes of this study were: (a) to determine the anaerobic threshold of cross-country skiers and biathlonists and (b) to evaluate the relationships among maximum oxygen uptake, anaerobic threshold, and the characteristics of skeletal muscle.

Materials and Methods

The subjects were 43 male cross-country skiers and 32 male biathlonists (range of ages: 12.2-29.7 years). Information on their training and their physical characteristics is presented in Table 1. The cross-country skiers were significantly taller and had trained significantly more than the biathlonists. The subjects gave their informed consent to participate in the measurements of this study.

Anaerobic threshold (AT) and maximum oxygen uptake ($max\dot{V}_{O_2}$) were determined on a bicycle ergometer (60 rpm). The beginning intensi-

Table 1—Characteristics and Training Data for the Subjects

Group characteristics	Cross-country skiers			Biathlonists		
	n	x̄	s	n	x̄	s
Physical:						
Age, years	43	18.1	1.6	32	18.7	4.2
Height, cm	43	178.8	5.5	32	175.6	6.8[a]
Weight, kg	43	69.9	6.3	32	64.6	9.5
Percentage of fat	43	10.7	2.4	32	11.4	2.4
Muscle, m. VL						
SDH nM × mg^{-1} prot × min^{-1}	43	13.9	2.2	30	11.2	2.2[a]
MDH nM × mg^{-1} prot × min^{-1}	43	1924.0	561.0	30	1812.0	299.0
CS nM × mg^{-1} prot × min^{-1}	43	145.0	32.0	29	149.0	38.0
LDH nM × mg^{-1} prot × min^{-1}	43	1403.0	524.0	30	1369.0	484.0
Percentage of ST fibers	43	54.0	10.2	32	51.7	7.4
Amount of training:						
km × year^{-1}	42	4143.0	932.0	17	3017.0	1375.0[a]

[a]Significant difference between groups, $p < .05$.

ty of exercise was 90 W. The power was increased every second minute by 30 W during the first 2-4 increments (according to the fitness level of the subject) and thereafter by 15 W every second minute until exhaustion, which occurred after about 20 to 25 min. of exercise. Ventilation ($\dot{V}E$), oxygen uptake ($\dot{V}_{O_2}$), and carbon dioxide production ($\dot{V}C_{O_2}$) were measured during the test for every 30-sec. period, using a semiautomated system. The highest sum of two successive 30-sec. determinations was taken as max$\dot{V}_{O_2}$.

To determine AT, VE and $\dot{V}C_{O_2}$ were plotted against the corresponding $\dot{V}_{O_2}$ and heart rate values (Figure 1). Departure from linearity in the respiratory responses was used as a criterion of anaerobic threshold. In the case of biathlonists, blood lactate concentration was determined after every second work load and the increase of blood lactate over about 4 mmoles was used together with the respiratory measurements. AT was determined visually and calculated in ml O_2 × kg^{-1} × min^{-1} (mlAT) and in percentage of max$\dot{V}_{O_2}$ (percentage of AT).

A muscle sample from the vastus lateralis muscle was obtained using the needle biopsy technique after the exercise test. Myosine ATPase staining was used to classify the muscle fibers to slow twitch (ST) or fast twitch (FT) types according to Gollnick et al. (1972). The following enzymatic activities were assayed from another portion of the muscle sample: SDH, MDH, CS, and LDH. The specific enzyme activities were

70   Rusko and Rahkila

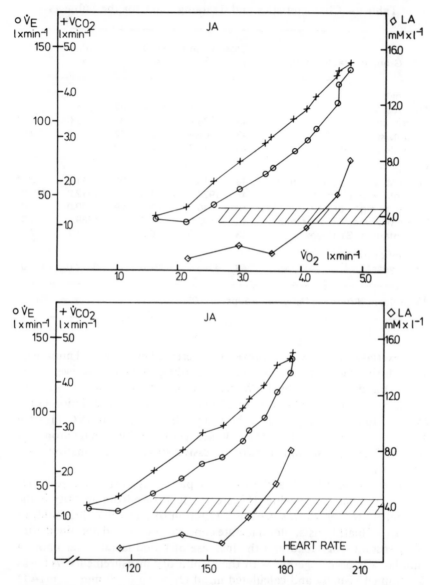

Figure 1—Example of anaerobic threshold (AT) determination. To determine AT, ventilation ($\dot{V}_E$), carbon dioxide production ($\dot{V}_{CO_2}$), and blood lactate (LA) values were plotted against corresponding oxygen uptake ($\dot{V}_{O_2}$) (upper figure) and heart rate values (lower figure).

referred to the protein content of the sample.

Table 2—Maximum and Anaerobic Threshold Values of the Subjects

Values	Cross-country skiers (n = 43)		Biathlonists (n = 32)	
	$\bar{x}$	s	$\bar{x}$	s
Maximum				
$\dot{V}_{O_2}$ l × min^{-1}	4.3	0.8	4.0	0.7
$\dot{V}_{O_2}$ ml × kg^{-1} × min^{-1}	62.0	8.0	61.0	5.0
Heart rate	191.0	10.0	192.0	8.0
Blood lactate, mM × 1^{-1}	9.4	2.0	10.2	1.9
Anaerobic threshold				
$\dot{V}_{O_2}$ l × min^{-1}	3.5	0.5	3.2	0.6[a]
$\dot{V}_{O_2}$ ml × kg^{-1} × min^{-1}	50.0	5.0	48.0	4.0
Percentage of max $\dot{V}_{O_2}$	80.0	6.0	78.0	4.0
Heart rate	175.0	10.0	175.0	8.0

[a]Significant difference between groups, $p < .05$.

Results

The mean max$\dot{V}_{O_2}$ of the subjects was 4.2 1 × min^{-1} or 62 ml × kg^{-1} × min^{-1}. The two groups did not differ from each other in max$\dot{V}_{O_2}$. The AT of the cross-country skiers (3.5 1 × min^{-1}) was significantly higher as compared with biathlonists (3.2 1 × min^{-1}) (Table 2). The heart rate corresponding to AT was 175 beats × min^{-1} in both groups. Table 1 shows that the muscle fiber composition and muscle enzyme activities of the groups were almost equal except for SDH activity, which was significantly higher in the cross-country skiers. The percentage of ST fibers showed no significant correlations with max$\dot{V}_{O_2}$ or anaerobic threshold. SDH activity correlated significantly with percentage of AT ($r = .24$, $p<.05$) and MDH activity with m1AT ($r = .27$, $p < .05$). None of the correlations between max$\dot{V}_{O_2}$ and the enzyme activities studied were statistically significant. Amount of training correlated significantly with SDH activity ($r = .29$, $p < .05$) and with m1AT ($r = .30$, $p<.01$), especially in the group of biathlonists ($r = .58$, $p < .05$ and $r = .73$, $p < .001$, respectively) (Figure 2). The correlation between max $\dot{V}_{O_2}$ and AT was highly significant (Figure 3). When the effect of age was removed by the partial correlation method, only minor changes in the correlations between variables were observed.

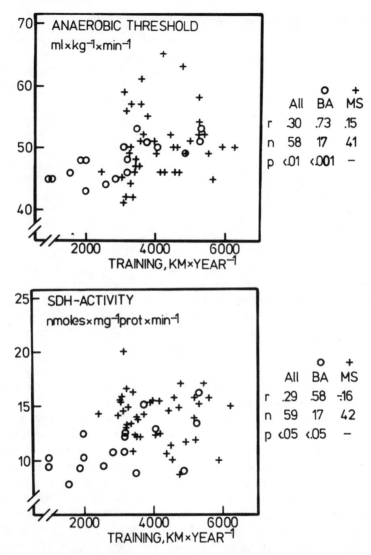

Figure 2—The relationships between the quantity of training and anaerobic threshold or succinate dehydrogenase (SDH) activity in biathlonists (BA) and male cross-country skiers (MS).

Discussion

The concept of anaerobic threshold has been adopted to describe the intensity of exercise or oxygen consumption at which a person can work for a prolonged period of time. According to European investigators, there might be two thresholds: the aerobic threshold at which blood lac-

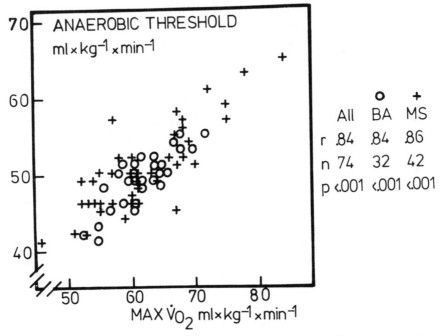

Figure 3—The relationship between maximum oxygen uptake (max$\dot{V}_{O_2}$) and anaerobic threshold in biathlonists (BA) and male cross-country skiers (MS).

tate starts to increase over resting (2 mmoles $\times$ 1^{-1}) values and the anaerobic threshold at which blood lactate increases over about 4 mmoles $\times$ $^{-1}$ (Kinderman et al., 1979; Mader et al., 1976). In our study, the 4 mmoles value of blood lactate was applied together with the respiratory measurements in biathlonists to determine the anaerobic threshold, and in most subjects, both thresholds were observed (Figure 1); however, in some cases only one threshold was found, and a simultaneous change both in respiratory and in blood lactate responses was not always observed. Furthermore, many subjects demonstrated a final abrupt increase in ventilation at very high intensities of exercise when blood lactate concentration was 6-8 mmoles. Perhaps due to the testing procedure, the preceding diet, or to some other factors, some subjects attained high blood lactate values at low intensities of exercise. These results might suggest that the 4 mmoles threshold value is not always valid and that perhaps endurance athletes are able to exercise for prolonged periods of time, even though their blood lactate is higher than 4 mmoles. Indeed, other investigators have shown that during distance-training the blood lactate of cross-country skiers may be 6-8 mmoles (Simon et al., 1979). Individual variation in maximal blood lactate concentration should also be taken into consideration as was suggested in a previous investigation on female cross-country skiers (Rusko et al., 1979). The abrupt increase in blood lactate concentration, together with the respiratory responses, might be more feasible than a rigid threshold level of 4 mmoles, and we do not feel very confident that respiratory responses without blood lactate measurements can be used for determination of AT.

According to these results, the anaerobic threshold correlated only slightly with the oxidative enzyme activities, and no significant correlations were observed between anaerobic threshold and percentage of ST fibers and LDH activity. In a previous study on female skiers, slightly higher correlations were found between the anaerobic threshold, on the one hand, and SDH and CS activity on the other, but the correlation between percentage of ST fibers and anaerobic threshold was not significant (Rusko et al., 1979). Amount of training correlated significantly both with SDH activity and anaerobic threshold, especially in the group of biathlonists (Figure 2). Furthermore, the cross-country skiers had trained more than the biathlonists and had higher SDH-activity and anaerobic threshold than the biathlonists. These results suggest that an influence of training existed both on SDH activity and on anaerobic threshold, and the slight correlations between enzyme activities and anaerobic threshold might have been determined by differences in the quantity of training. Consequently, the oxidative and glycolytic capacities of the muscles seem to contribute only slightly to the anaerobic threshold, and the contribution of other factors might be of equal or even of greater importance.

One explanation for the onset of metabolic acidosis might be an imbalance between glycolysis and the pyruvate transport into or utilization in the mitochondria. On the other hand, a high correlation between maximum oxygen uptake and the anaerobic threshold suggests that the same factors might have influenced both of the variables. These factors could be related to the oxygen transport (e.g., capillarization) and the oxygen supply to the working muscles. Although it was assumed that the oxygen supply is adequate at anaerobic threshold, the lack of oxygen in the contracting muscle fibers could also explain the observed onset of metabolic acidosis.

Acknowledgments

The able assistance of Miss Ursula Salonen, Miss Eija Tulonen, Mr. Teuvo Ylikoski, and Mr. Matti Virtanen is gratefully acknowledged.

This study was supported by grants 8851/78/77 and 8333/78/78 from the Ministry of Education, Finland and a grant from the Finnish Central Sports Federation.

References

Bergh, U., Thorstensson, A., Sjodin, B., Hulten, B., Piehl, K., and Karlsson, J. 1978. Maximal oxygen uptake and muscle fiber types in trained and untrained humans. *Med. Sci. Sports* **10**:151-154.

Gollnick, P.D., Armstrong, R.B., Saubert, C.W.IV, Piehl, K., and Saltin, B. 1972. Enzyme activity and fiber composition in skeletal muscle of untrained and trained men. *J. Appl. Physiol.* **33**:312-319.

Holloszy, J. 1967. Biochemical adaptations in muscle. Effects of exercise on mitochondrial oxygen uptake and respiratory enzyme activity in skeletal muscle. *J. Biol. Chem.* **242**:2278-2282.

Kinderman, W., Simon, G., and Keul, J. 1979. The significance of the aerobic-anaerobic transition for the determination of work load intensities during endurance training. *Eur. J. Appl. Physiol.* **42**:25-34.

Mader, A., Liesen, H., Heck, H., Philippi, H., Rost, R., Schurch, P., and Hollmann, W. 1976. Zur Beurteilung des sportartspezifischen Ausdauerleitungsfahigkeit im Labor. (Evaluation of specific endurance capacity in the laboratory.) *Sportarzt und Sportmedizin* **27**:80-88.

Rusko, H., Havu, M., and Karvinen, E. 1978. Aerobic performance capacity in athletes. *Eur. J. Appl. Physiol.* **38**:151-159.

Rusko, H., Rahkila, P., and Karvinen, E. 1979. Anaerobic threshold, skeletal muscle enzymes and fiber composition in young female cross-country skiers. *Acta Physiol. Scand.* (in press).

Simon, G., Huber, G., Dickhuth, H.-H., and Keul, J. 1979. Herzfrequenzen und Lactatverhalten von Skilanglaufern bei Laufbandergometrie und wettkampf-spezifischem Training. (Response of heart rate and blood lactate during tread-mill exercise and specific training of cross-country skiers) *Leistungssport* **9**:117-120.

Weltman, A., Katch, V., Sady, S., and Freedson. 1978. Onset of metabolic acidosis (anaerobic threshold) as a criterion measure of submaximum fitnesss. *Res. Quart.* **49**:218-227.

Muscle Fibers, Exercise, and Training

Muscle Fiber Type Distribution in Trained and Untrained Muscles of Athletes

Per Tesch, Jan Karlsson, and **Bertil Sjödin**
Karolinska Hospital, Sweden

During the past decade, various investigations have been designed to examine muscle fiber composition in different athletic groups. It is obvious that endurance-trained athletes possess a high percentage of slow twitch (ST, type I) fibers in the trained muscle (Costill et al., 1976; Gollnick et al., 1972, Komi et al., 1977), whereas strength-trained and power-trained athletes tend to exhibit an opposite pattern (Komi et al., 1977; Thorstensson et al., 1977). Still the question exists of whether this pattern reflects a genetic selection of individuals or is due to a local training-induced adaptation. Until recently, investigations based on histochemical stainings for myofibrillar ATPase have failed to demonstrate changes in the percentage of the two main muscle fiber types as a result of endurance (Gollnick et al., 1973), sprint (Thorstensson et al., 1975), and strength (Thorstennson et al., 1976) training. However, Jansson et al. (1978) in a longitudinal study found evidence for a possible change in muscle fiber type composition as a result of a change in training regimen. Thus, a higher percentage of ST fibers was demonstrated in m. vastus lateralis after aerobic distance running in comparison with anaerobic high intensive running. To add further information concerning the possibility of a muscle fiber type adaptation to training, trained as well as untrained muscles of successful athletes were studied.

Subjects and Methods

Muscle fiber type distribution in m. vastus lateralis and m. deltoideus were examined in 58 subjects, a control group of physically active, but not specifically trained, physical education students ($n = 12$) and a study

Table 1—Anthropometric Characteristics of the Subject Groups

Group	n	Age (yr.)	Height (cm)	Weight (kg)
European handball players	8	26 (21-32)	186 (180-194)	81 (76-91)
Ice hockey players	8	24 (20-29)	181 (176-184)	75 (72-80)
Kayak paddlers	8	22 (20-28)	183 (179-196)	76 (71-83)
Middle and long distance runners	8	25 (22-30)	180 (174-185)	68 (62-73)
Water skiers	6	23 (18-30)	181 (178-185)	74 (71-81)
Wrestlers	8	23 (19-30)	173 (160-184)	75 (60-86)
Physical education students	12	21 (19-26)	181 (174-185)	72 (66-80)

Note. Values are means (ranges).

group of European handball players ($n = 8$), ice hockey players ($n = 8$), kayak paddlers ($n = 8$), middle and long distance runners ($n = 8$), water skiers ($n = 6$), and wrestlers ($n = 8$) (Table 1).

Most of the athletes were members of Swedish national teams and participants in Olympic Games or World Championships. Muscle biopsies were obtained during or following the competitive seasons. Cross-sections of tissue samples were histochemically stained for myofibrillar ATPase after preincubation at pH 10.3 (Padykula and Herman, 1955). Muscle fibers were identified either as slow twitch (ST, type I) or as fast twitch (FT, type II) fibers according to Engel (1962). Muscle fiber type distribution was expressed as percentage of ST fibers. Tissue samples from kayak paddlers were further examined for identification of subgroups of FT fibers (Brooke and Kaiser, 1970).

Results

Values (mean, range) for muscle fiber type distribution for the different athletic groups are presented in Table 2. Ice hockey players, kayak paddlers, and wrestlers demonstrated a significantly lower percentage of ST fibers in m. vastus lateralis as compared with m. deltoideus. The opposite pattern (i.e., a lower percentage of ST fibers in m. deltoideus) was established in runners, whereas no significant difference between trained and untrained muscles (i.e., 50% ST in m. deltoideus and 43% ST in m. vastus lateralis) was present in physical education students. In comparison with the latter group only kayak paddlers and middle and long distance runners demonstrated a significantly ($p < 0.01$) different muscle fiber type distribution. Thus, in the deltoid muscle of kayak paddlers, a mean value of 73% ST fibers was found, and the vastus lateralis muscle

Table 2—Mean values (ranges) for Muscle Fiber Type Distribution
(Percentage of ST) in M. Vastus Lateralis and M. Deltoideus
of Different Subject Groups

Group	Percentage of ST m. vastus lateralis	Percentage of ST m. deltoideus
Handball players	51 (35-74)	61 (45-72)
Ice hockey players	42 (17-58)	58 (38-81)[a]
Kayak paddlers	41 (25-56)	73 (54-82)[a]
Middle and long distance runners	67 (55-73)	50 (38-66)[a]
Water skiers	52 (38-78)	59 (37-80)
Wrestlers	47 (22-63)	61 (38-87)[a]
Physical education students	43 (26-59)	50 (33-64)

Note. [a]Intraindividual differences $= p < 0.05$.

of runners averaged 67% ST fibers. The "untrained" muscle of kayak paddlers (m. vastus lateralis) and runners (m. deltoideus) did not differ significantly from values obtained from the other groups (Fig. 1). In the deltoid muscle of kayak paddlers, all FT fibers studied (27%) were rated as FTa fibers, whereas in m. vastus lateralis 29% of the sample were found to be FTb fibers (41% ST, 30% FTa).

Discussion

In agreement with previous studies (Costill et al., 1976; Gollnick et al., 1972; Komi et al., 1977), the present investigation demonstrates that endurance-trained muscles of athletes are composed of a high percentage of ST fibers. The main finding of the present study is the observed difference in fiber type composition of endurance-trained and untrained muscles of the same individuals. This pattern is most obvious when comparing the deltoid and vastus lateralis muscles in kayak paddlers with those of middle and long distance runners.

In contrast with other athletic groups studied, these events actively involve one of the muscles, whereas the other muscle remains metabolically inactive. The value obtained for m. vastus lateralis of middle and long distance runners is comparable to earlier findings (Forsberg et al., 1976). The deltoid muscles of successful kayak paddlers have been investigated previously. In agreement with the present findings, Tesch et al. (1976) and Rusko (1976) demonstrated a high percentage of ST fibers. Gollnick et al. (1972) reported lower values, comparable to the value obtained

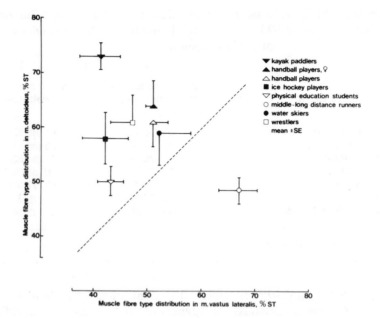

Figure 1—The relationship between muscle fiber type distribution (percentage of ST) in m. vastus lateralis and m. deltoideus. Values are mean (± SE). Dotted line denotes "line of identity." The value for a group of national elite female handball players ($n = 5$) is also included.

from a group of former world-class kayak paddlers (Tesch et al., 1976). In the study by Gollnick et al., (1972), however, biopsy samplings were taken during the off-season (Piehl, personal communication), and Tesch et al. (1976) studied athletes who withdrew from strenuous training at least 2 years before examination. It can be questioned whether muscle fiber type distribution in the inactive state reflects the potential of the active muscle. Whether or not this is true in the latter group it was possible to relate the preferred racing distance to fiber type distribution. Neither in the present study nor in the study on active kayak paddlers by Tesch et al. (1976) was such a relationship present. Hence, irrespective of preferred racing distance (performance time approximately 2-45 min.) kayak paddlers demonstrated the same muscle fiber type distribution in m. deltoideus. It is of interest to note that the muscle fiber type distribution pattern of m. vastus lateralis tends to reflect performance capacity; thus, the three most successful short distance paddlers had an average of 32% ST fibers in m. vastus lateralis. Interpreting the accumulated information from examination of kayak paddlers, it seems reasonable to suggest that muscle fiber composition is under the influence of hereditary factors (Komi and Karlsson, 1979) but that specific training, at least temporarily, can induce changes in muscle fiber composition (Jansson et al., 1978) as a result of either fiber splitting or transformation processes. The fact that only runners demonstrate a significantly higher percentage of ST fibers in m. vastus lateralis as compared with m. deltoideus does not contradict this interpretation.

References

Brooke, M.H., and Kaiser, K. 1970. Muscle fiber types: How many and what kind? *Arch. Neurol.* **23**:369-379.

Costill, D.L., Daniels, J., Evans, W., Fink, W., Kraehenbuhl, G., and Saltin, B. 1976. Skeletal muscle enzymes and fiber composition in male and female track athletes. *J. Appl. Physiol.* **40**:149-154.

Engel, W.K. 1962. The essentiality of histo- and cytochemical studies of skeletal muscle in the investigation of neuromuscular disease. *Neurology.* **12**:778-794.

Forsberg, A., Tesch, P., Sjodin, B., Thorstensson, A., and Karlsson, J. 1976. Skeletal muscle fibers and athletic performance. In: Paavo V. Komi (ed.), *Biomechanics* **V**, pp. 112-117. University Park Press, Baltimore.

Gollnick, P.D., Armstrong, R.B., Saltin, B., Saubert, IV, C.W., Sembrowich, W.L., and Shepherd, R.E. 1973. Effect of training on enzyme activity and fiber composition of human skeletal muscle. *J. Appl. Physiol.* **34**:107-111.

Gollnick, P.D., Armstrong, R.B., Saubert, IV, C.W., Piehl, K., and Saltin, B. 1972. Enzyme activity and fiber composition in skeletal muscle of untrained and trained men. *J. Appl. Physiol.* **33**:312-319.

Jansson, E., Sjodin, B., and Tesch, P. 1978. Changes in muscle fibre type distribution in man after physical training. A sign of fibre type transformation? *Acta Physiol. Scand.* **104**:235-237.

Komi, P.V., and Karlsson, J. 1979. Physical performance, skeletal muscle enzyme activities, and fibre types in monozygous and dizygous twins of both sexes. *Acta Physiol. Scand.,* Suppl. **462**.

Komi, P.V., Rusko, H., Vos, J., and Vihko, V. 1977. Anaerobic performance capacity in athletes. *Acta Physiol. Scand.* **100**:107-114.

Padykula, H.A., and Herman, E. 1955. The specificity of the histochemical method for adenosine triphosphatase. *J. Histochem. Cytochem.* **3**:170-195.

Rusko, H. 1976. Physical Performance Characteristics in Finnish Athletes. Ph.D. dissertation, University of Jyväskylä, Jyväskylä, Finland.

Tesch, P., Piehl, K., Wilson, G., and Karlsson, J. 1976. Physiological investigations of Swedish elite canoe competitors. *Med. Sci. Sports* **8**:214-218.

Thorstensson, A., Hulten, B., von Dobeln, W., and Karlsson, J. 1976. Effect of strength training on enzyme activities and fibre characteristics in human skeletal muscle. *Acta Physiol. Scand.* **96**:392-398.

Thorstensson, A., Larsson, L., Tesch, P., and Karlsson, J. 1977. Muscle strength and fiber composition in athletes and sedentary men. *Med. Sci. Sports* **9**:26-30.

Thorstensson, A., Sjodin, B., and Karlsson, J. 1975. Enzyme activities and muscle strength after "sprint training" in man. *Acta Physiol. Scand.* **94**:313-318.

Running Performance and Muscle Fiber Types

Rickard Schéle and **Peter Kaiser**
National Defense Research Institute
and Karolinska Hospital, Stockholm, Sweden

It is well documented that long distance runners have a high percentage of slow twitch fibers (Costill et al., 1976). No clearcut pattern has been demonstrated for sprinters in terms of muscle fiber types; they only tend to have a higher percentage of fast twitch fibers than a normal population (Bergh et al., 1978). In most studies, however, a significant difference exists between long distance runners and sprinters in terms of muscle fiber composition (Costill et al., 1976; Gollnick et al., 1972; Komi et al., 1977; Thorstensson et al., 1977). In a series of recent studies where short-term performance has been studied in laboratory experiments with different procedures, it has been possible to demonstrate a positive relationship between performance capacity and the percentage of fast twitch fibers (Bar-Or et al., 1980; Thorstensson, 1976). To provide further information concerning this relationship, a study was undertaken to examine in the same individuals both sprint running and long distance running performance and to evaluate different physiological characteristics which might be of importance.

Subjects and Methods

Thirty-nine subjects participated in the study. All were physically trained and participated in regular training programs for running. They were not specially trained for the 100 m dash or marathon running nor were they elite competitors. In 21 subjects, muscle biopsies were obtained from the vastus lateralis muscle for fiber typing (for references, see Thorstensson, 1976). The muscle fibers were classified as slow twitch (ST) and fast twitch (FT) (type I or II fibers, respectively). The running tests were performed over the following distances: 40 m (flying start),

Table 1—Some Characteristics of the Subjects

Group characteristics	$\bar{x}$	SD	Range
Age (years)	23.7	5.1	16-35
Weight (kg)	69.2	5.3	60.2-79.4
Height (mm)	1807.0	51.0	1732-1925
Muscle fiber composition (percentage of FT)	46.2	15.4	14-74
Running speed (m × s^{-1})			
40 m	8.1	0.5	7.2-9.1
300 m	7.2	0.4	6.4-7.9
2000 m	5.2	0.4	4.4-5.9

Note. n = 21

300 m, and 2,000 m. The muscle power of the subjects was tested in the laboratory with repeated isokinetic knee extensions according to Thorstensson (1976) and with the Wingate muscle power test (Bar-Or, 1980). Maximal oxygen uptake ($\dot{V}_{O_2}$ max) during running was assessed using the Douglas bag procedure as described by Saltin and Astrand (1967) for 18 additional subjects.

Results

Anthropometric data, muscle fiber composition, running speed, and some laboratory data are presented in Table 1.

Performance capacity when running 40 m was positively correlated to the percentage of FT fibers in the vastus lateralis muscle ($r=0.73$) (Figure 1). The opposite pattern was present for running performance at 2,000 m; i.e., the lower the percentage of FT fibers the better the performance ($r=-0.60$) (Figure 2). Running performance at 300 m was not significantly correlated to muscle fiber composition.

The two laboratory tests for muscle power, the isokinetic test and the Wingate test, showed positive correlations to performance at 300 m when the measures for average peak torque and average power, respectively, were applied. The peak torque decrease of the isokinetic test was correlated to performance at 2,000 m ($r=-0.54$). Thus, the subjects who fatigued more in the isokinetic test had a slower running time. In the additional 18 subjects, a negative relationship was present between maximal oxygen uptake and the muscle fiber composition expressed as percentage of FT fibers, i.e., the more ST fibers the higher the maximal oxygen uptake (Figure 3).

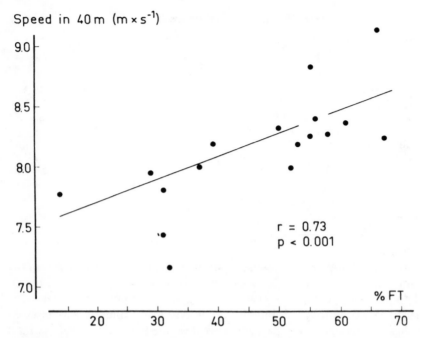

Figure 1—Relationship between speed in a 40 m run and muscle fiber composition (percentage of fast twitch fibers).

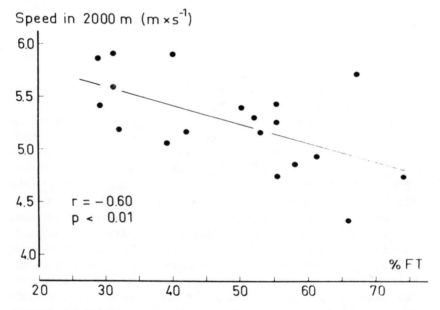

Figure 2—Relationship between speed in a 2,000 m run and muscle fiber composition (percentage of fast twitch fibers).

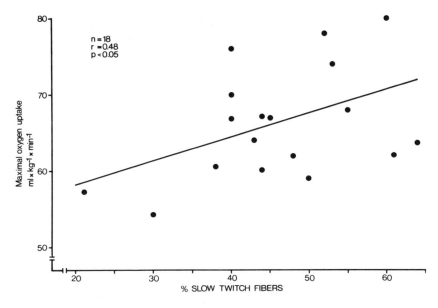

Figure 3—Relationship between maximal oxygen uptake ($\dot{V}_{O_2}$ max, ml $\times$ kg^{-1} $\times$ min^{-1}) and muscle fiber composition (percentage of slow twitch fibers).

Discussion

It should be emphasized that the subjects were recruited because of their preference for either long distance or short distance running; however, the short distance runners also trained for distances corresponding to 1,000-2,000 m. The group which was examined for maximal oxygen uptake competed at distances ranging from 400 m to 10,000 m. Because of the criteria for selection of the subjects, the correlations obtained do not necessarily reflect the degree of correlation in a normal population. It seems reasonable, however, to assume that the correlations will indicate some of the physiological features of significance for performance in the trained state and might even be indicative of training potentials in sedentary subjects.

It seems reasonable to conclude that muscle fiber composition is of importance for short-term performance (Figure 1) as well as for endurance type exercise (Figure 2) but of minor importance for "intermediate-term" performance. The correlation between endurance performance and muscle fiber composition (Figure 2) is evidently due to the fact that muscle fiber composition in trained subjects at least partly determines the maximal oxygen uptake (Figure 3, Bergh et al., 1978; Costill et al., 1976).

The fast twitch fibers have a metabolic profile which favors fast utilization of phosphagen stores as well as high glycogenolytic activity. The slow twitch fibers, on the other hand, have a profile in favor of combustion and, thus, fat utilization. No difference or very small differences exist between the two main fiber types in terms of glycogen stores in the resting, well-fed state; but large differences exist in terms of fat depots between the two fiber types (Essen, 1978). In addition to these metabolic differences, differences exist in terms of the mechanical behavior and the motoric control (Komi et al., 1981).

To what extent these significant features for physical performance are determined by genetic factors, training, sport activity, and nutrition during adolescence is still unknown; however, Komi and Karlsson (1979) demonstrated that muscle fiber compositon is to a great extent genetically determined. Jansson et al. (1978) showed that training can change the muscle fiber composition. It seems reasonable to assume that performance characteristics, as evaluated in the present study, are influenced by all these factors and that part of the influence is mediated by the muscle fiber composition.

Acknowledgments

The study was supported by grants from the Swedish Medical Research Council (No.4251) and the Research Council of the Swedish Sports Federation.

References

Bar-Or, O. 1980. A new anaerobic capacity test—characteristics and applications. *Med. Esporte Porto Alegre.* **5**:73-82.

Bar-Or, O., Dotan, R., Inbar, O., Rothstein, A., Karlsson, J., and Tesch, P. 1980. Anaerobic capacity and muscle fibre type distribution in man. *Int. J. Sports Med.* **1**:82-85.

Bergh, U., Thorstensson, A., Sjodin, B., Hulten, B., Piehl, K., and Karlsson, J. 1978. Maximal oxygen uptake and muscle fiber types in trained and untrained humans. *Med. Sci. Sports* **10**:151-154.

Costill, D.L., Daniels, J., Evans, W., Fink, W., Krahenbuhl, G., and Saltin, B. 1976. Skeletal muscle enzymes and fiber composition in male and female track athletes. *J. Appl. Physiol.* **40**:149-154.

Essen, B. 1978. Studies on the regulation of metabolism in human skeletal muscle using intermittent exercise as an experimental model. *Acta Physiol. Scand.,* Suppl. **454**.

Gollnick, P.D., Armstrong, R.B., Saubert, C.W. IV, Piehl, K., and Saltin, B. 1972. Enzyme activity and fiber composition in skeletal muscle of untrained and trained men. *J. Appl. Physiol.* **33**:312-319.

Jansson, E., Sjodin, B., and Tesch, P. 1978. Changes in muscle fibre type distribution after physical training. A sign of fibre type transformation? *Acta Physiol. Scand.* **104**:235-237.

Komi, P.V., Ito, A., Sjodin, B., and Karlsson, J. 1981. Muscle metabolism, lactate breaking point, and biomechanical features of endurance running. *Int. J. Sports Med.* **2**:148-153.

Komi, P.V., and Karlsson, J. 1979. Physical performance, skeletal muscle enzyme activities, and fibre types in monozygous and dizygous twins of both sexes. *Acta Physiol. Scand.,* Suppl. **462**.

Komi, P.V., Rusko, H., Vos, J., and Vihko, V. 1977. Anaerobic performance capacity in athletes. *Acta Physiol. Scand.* **100**:107-114.

Saltin, B., and Astrand, P.-O. 1967. Maximal oxygen uptake in athletes. *J. Appl. Physiol.* **23**(3):353-358.

Thorstensson, A. 1976. Muscle strength, fibre types and enzyme activities in man. *Acta Physiol. Scand.,* Suppl. **443**.

Thorstensson, A., Larsson, L., Tesch, P., and Karlsson, J. 1977. Muscle strength and fiber composition in athletes and sedentary men. *Med. Sci. Sports* **9**:26-30.

Effects of Heavy Resistance and Explosive-type Strength Training Methods on Mechanical, Functional, and Metabolic Aspects of Performance

P.V. Komi, H. Suominen and **E. Heikkinen**
University of Jyväskylä, Finland

J. Karlsson and **P. Tesch**
Karolinska Hospital, Stockholm, Sweden

One question concerning strength training is the specificity of training programs. Improvement of those attributes of the neuromuscular function which have been trained may simultaneously weaken or retard the development of other performance characteristics. The present study was undertaken to examine this hypothesis with two kinds of strength training regimens: heavy weight training and training with lighter loads and explosive-type jumps.

Methods

The training program covered a 16-week period during late fall and early winter (Figure 1). During this period, the subjects were also allowed to participate in other physical activities. None of these activities was competitive in nature and their intensity level and duration were negligible when compared with the prescribed strength training programs.

Two specific training programs were used: (a) conventional heavy weight training (weight training group, WT), where primarily the lower extremity (leg extensors) muscles were trained with high-intensity barbell loads and (b) light weights with fast contraction and explosive-type jumps (jump training, JT). The programs were run parallel in two physical education institutes. The subjects were students in the respective institutes. The two training groups were guided by qualified coaches, who instructed the subjects, kept records of their training, and handled the

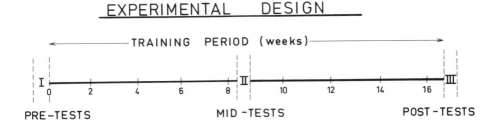

EXPERIMENTAL   DESIGN

← TRAINING PERIOD (weeks) →

I ├────┼────┼────┼────┼── II ├────┼────┼────┼────┤ III
0   2   4   6   8   10   12   14   16

PRE-TESTS   MID-TESTS   POST-TESTS

STRENGTH   TRAINING   GROUPS

HEAVY   WEIGHT   TRAINING   LIGHTER   WEIGHTS   AND
                                   EXPLOSIVE   JUMPS

(WT , N = 10)   (JT , N = 8)

16 weeks   16 weeks
3 times a week   3 times a week

MEASUREMENTS

ANTHROPOMETRICS	PERFORMANCE	MUSCLE BIOPSY
WEIGHT	RUNNING VELOCITY	FIBER DISTRIBUTION
HEIGHT	VERTICAL JUMP	ST
FAT % AND KG	MUSCULAR POWER	FT
SKELETAL WEIGHT	ISOMETRIC STRENGTH	FIBER DIAMETERS
THIGH GIRTH	STRENGTH ENDURANCE	ENZYME ACTIVITIES
		$Mg^{2+}ATPase$
		MK, CPK,

Figure 1—Summary of experimental design; training groups and variables measured. For methodological references of anthropometric measurements, running velocity, muscular power, isometric strength, and enzyme activities, see Komi and Karlsson (1979). Other references: Vertical jump performed with preliminary counter-movement (Komi and Bosco, 1978); strength endurance at 0.5 × Po (Viitasalo and Komi, 1978); muscle biopsies were taken from the vastus lateralis muscle according to Bergstrom (1962); fiber type distribution (Gollnick et al., 1972); lesser fiber diameter (Larsson, 1978).

possible overtraining syndromes. In both groups, the training was undertaken three times a week for a period of 16 weeks. The JT and WT groups were composed of 10 and 8 subjects, respectively, who completed the entire training program. Two and three subjects, respectively, were originally signed up but were eliminated from the study because periodic injuries and infections reduced their number of training sessions by more than 20%. Figure 1 gives a detailed summary of the experimental design and of the variables measured.

Table 1—Means (±S.D.) of the Selected Performance Variables in the Two Training Groups

Groups	Tests	Weight (kg)	Total leg force (N)	Strength endurance (s)	Vertical jump (cm)	Running velocity (V_v, m/s)
Jump training ($n = 10$)	I	71.6 ± 13.9	3,271 ± 65	67.0 ± 21.6	45.7 ± 5.4	1.58 ± 0.09
	II	72.6 ± 13.1	3,906 ± 95	73.2 ± 18.9	39.7 ± 3.3	1.64 ± 0.14
	III	72.5 ± 12.9	3,851 ± 102	72.7 ± 22.0	47.3 ± 7.3	1.69 ± 0.13
Weight training ($n = 8$)	I	75.1 ± 3.7	3,327 ± 48	67.8 ± 16.0	48.0 ± 4.8	1.50 ± 0.11
	II	77.6 ± 7.9	3,983 ± 74	69.1 ± 16.7	47.5 ± 4.8	1.56 ± 0.10
	III	77.2 ± 7.5	4,016 ± 87	73.1 ± 11.9	47.9 ± 4.8	1.64 ± 0.09

Table 2—Means (±S.D.) of the Muscle Biopsy (m. vastus lateralis) Variables in the Two Training Groups

Groups	Percentage of ST fibers	FT fiber diameter (mm × 10^{-3})	ST fiber diameter (mm × 10^{-3})	Mg^{2+} ATPase (moles × g^{-1} × min^{-1} × 10^{-6})	Myokinase (moles × g^{-1} × min^{-1} × 10^{-6})	CPK (moles × g^{-1} × min^{-1} × 10^{-4})
Jump training (n = 10)						
I	50.9 ± 14.7	1.28 ± 0.15	1.30 ± 0.16	7.10 ± 3.02	1.63 ± 0.34	3.04 ± 0.36
II	47.5 ± 1.24	1.39 ± 0.26	1.33 ± 0.20	6.80 ± 2.83	1.64 ± 0.37	3.11 ± 0.70
III	55.2 ± 1.28	1.32 ± 0.23	1.28 ± 0.26	6.67 ± 2.33	1.97 ± 0.41	3.07 ± 0.76
Weight training (n = 8)						
I	44.4 ± 14.1	1.23 ± 0.07	1.18 ± 0.09	5.66 ± 2.50	1.66 ± 0.33	3.06 ± 0.29
II	48.9 ± 14.9	1.33 ± 0.17	1.26 ± 0.14	5.91 ± 2.16	1.78 ± 0.21	3.20 ± 0.56
III	46.6 ± 11.9	1.44 ± 0.18	1.40 ± 0.15	6.20 ± 2.61	1.73 ± 0.28	3.13 ± 0.82

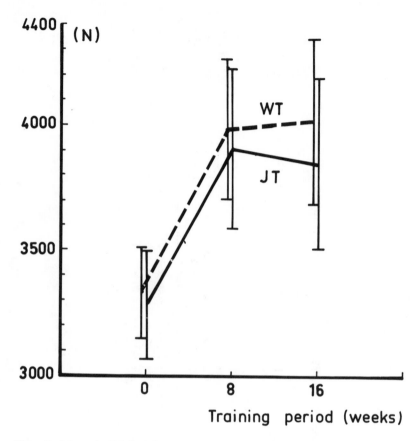

Figure 2—Means (±S.D.) of the maximum isometric extension force of both legs during the 16 weeks of strength training. WT—heavy weight training group; JT—explosive-type jump training group.

Results and Discussion

Tables 1 and 2 present the results of the major performance and muscle biopsy variables, respectively. No changes were observed in the anthropometric variables during training.

Performance Variables

Both the heavy weight training and explosive-type jump training improved isometric strength in a similar way, although the JT group attained its maximal value after only 8 weeks of training (Figure 2; Table 1). The average increases in strength during the entire training period of

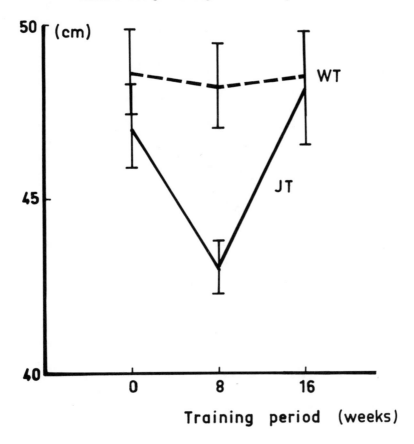

Figure 3—Maximum height of rise of center of gravity in the vertical jump measured on three different occasions during the 16-week training period. For symbols WT and JT, see Figure 1. The jumping was performed on the force-platform with allowance for preparatory counter-movement. Hands were kept on the hips throughout the jump.

16 weeks were 20 ± 2.0 (SD)% and 17.4 ± 2.5%, respectively, for weight training and jump training groups.

The vertical jump test performed on the force platform (Komi and Bosco, 1978) was used to examine changes in the "explosive-type dynamic leg strength" during training. The results were markedly different between the two groups. The subjects in WT group maintained a similar jumping height in all three tests, whereas the JT group decreased its performance by an average of 9% during the first half of training ($p < .001$). This group was, however, able to regain its initial jumping height during the second 8-week period of training (Figure 3). A similar effect of "explosive jump" training has earlier been reported for volleyball players (Komi et al., 1978).

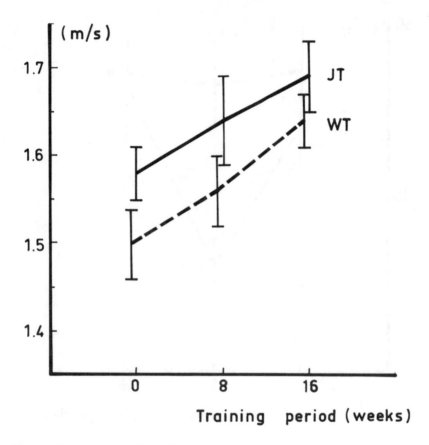

Figure 4—Improvement of the vertical running velocity in the two training groups during the 16-week heavy weight (WT) and explosive jump (JT) training.

Vertical running velocity, as obtained with the Margaria test (Margaria et al., 1966), increased linearly and the training effects were similar in both groups (Table 1; Figure 4). The subjects in jumping training had higher initial values of the vertical velocity (1.58 ± 0.09 m/s vs. 1.50 ± 0.11 m/s; $p<.01$). The final values (1.69 ± 0.13 and 1.64 ± 0.09, respectively for JT and WT) were also different ($p<.05$). Changes in muscular power, which were calculated from the vertical running velocity (Komi et al., 1973), were in accordance with improvements in running velocity.

Muscle endurance capacity was tested by means of recording the maintenance time of a force corresponding to 50% of the initial maximal isometric leg strength. Each subject was instructed to maintain this force level till exhaustion in Tests I, II, and III. The WT group showed almost a linear increase during the entire 16-week training period and changed its endurance time from 67.8 ± 16.0 s to 73.1 ± 11.9 s (Table 1). The JT group improved its strength endurance during the first half of training (from 67.0 ± 21.6 to 73.2 ± 18.9 s); thereafter, the endurance time stayed nearly the same.

Muscle Biopsy Variables

Muscle fiber composition as expressed in percentage of slow twitch fibers (percentage of ST, Table 2) showed no change in either group during training. Muscle fiber diameters changed in the WT group, where both fiber types hypertrophied by 17% (FT fibers) and 19% (ST fibers) (Figure 5). In the JT group, the initial fiber diameters of both types were slightly larger ($p < .05$ for ST fibers; n.s. for FT fibers) than in the WT group. The final values in the JT group were, however, much below those in the WT group ($p < .01$; see Table 2), and therefore no training effect could be seen in the JT group.

With the exception of myokinase activity none of the enzymes studied showed a training-induced change. Myokinase appeared to be affected by the training regimens in differential ways (Figure 6). WT appeared to have an increase (n.s.) in myokinase activity during the first 8 weeks, but this increase vanished during the second part of the training period. The JT group, on the other hand, showed no change during the first half of the training period but a 20% increase during the second half (see also Table 2).

Other Observations

Although the training programs demonstrated differential effects with respect to muscle fiber diameters and myokinase activity, no significant differences were observed between the two regimens when physiological and muscle biopsy variables were intercorrelated. For this reason, the data were pooled and the most significant relationships identified for the initial test. During this test, measurements were taken from an additional 14 subjects, who took no part in training. Figures 7 and 8 present results from these comparisons.

As could be expected from earlier results (Hulten et al., 1975; Viitasalo and Komi, 1978) isometric endurance time was positively related to percentage of ST fibers (Figure 7a). Similarly, and in accordance with previous observations (Bosco and Komi, 1979), the height of rise of center of gravity in the vertical jump test was higher when the percentage of ST was smaller (Figure 7b).

As already noted, only the heavy weight training program caused hypertrophy of the muscle fiber types. In pretests, the subjects showed a good relationship between FT and ST fiber diameters with two exceptions (Figure 8). These two subjects had previously participated in

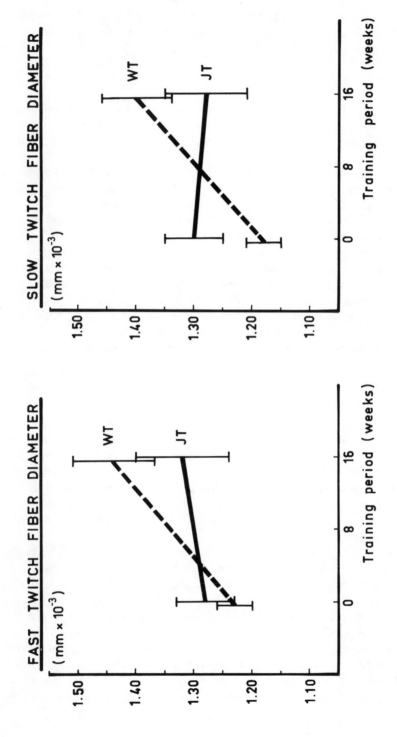

Figure 5—Means (±S.D.) for the lesser diameter of fast and slow twitch muscle fibers in the beginning and at the end of 16 weeks of training; WT—heavy weight training; JT—explosive type jump training.

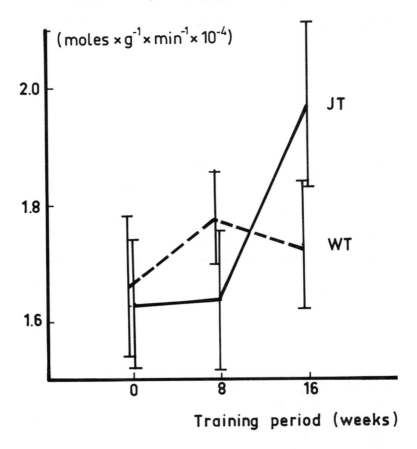

Figure 6—Myokinase activity in the two strength training groups during the 16 weeks of training.

specialized training regimens, one as a shot putter and the other as an endurance runner. Probably for that reason, their values differed from each other and from the other subjects in Figure 8. This observation seems to agree with that of Edstrom and Ekblom (1972) in that athletes engaged in weight lifting exercises for several years have slightly bigger FT than ST fibers; however, those subjects who belonged to the weight training group in the present study had a hypertrophy response which was similar in both types of muscle fibers.

In conclusion, diversified strength training programs in terms of heavy loads compared to low-resistance jumping exercises of 16-weeks' duration had similar training effects on a number of performance characteristics. The major differences could be seen primarily in two parameters: (a) increase in muscle fiber diameter of both FT and ST

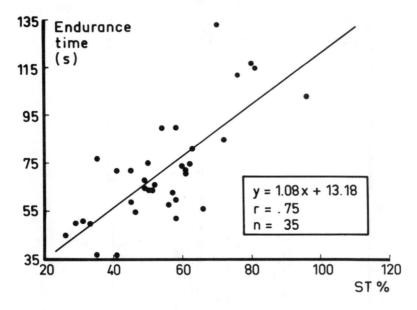

Figure 7a—Relationship between isometric endurance time and percentage of distribution of slow twitch fibers (percentage of ST).

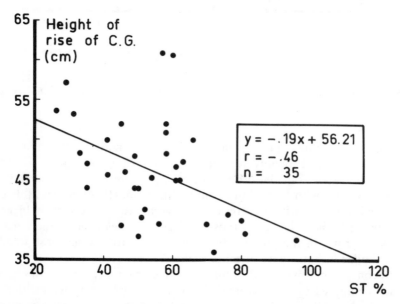

Figure 7b—Relationship between the height of rise of center of gravity (vertical jump) and percentage of distribution of slow twitch fibers (percentage of ST). Comparisons were made from the pretest measurements, where the total number of subjects was 34.

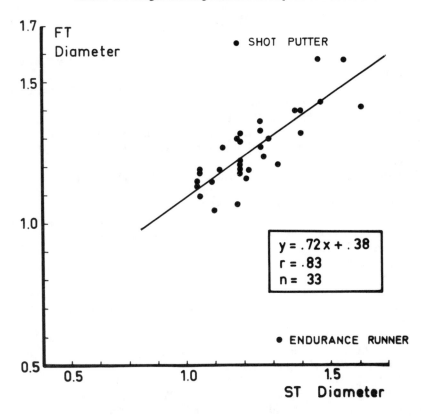

Figure 8—Relationship between the lesser diameter (mm $\times 10^{-3}$) of fast twitch (FT) and slow twitch (ST) fibers ($n = 34$). The two designated points represent subjects who had been engaged in special training for several years.

fibers, which occurred only in the heavy weight training group and (b) increased activity of the enzyme myokinase, which took place in the jump training group. Weight training as used in the present study was carried out with slow muscle contractions. Good reason exists, therefore, to believe that both fiber types were very active during contractions and were subjected to hypertrophy. In contrast, jump training seemed to induce qualitative changes as manifested by the increased myokinase activity. This increase occurred simultaneously when the subjects in jump training regained their vertical jumping performance, which was markedly reduced during the first 8 weeks of training. It is possible that these two changes are linked, although the present data warrant no further predictions.

References

Bergstrom, J. 1962. Muscle electrolytes in man. *Scand. J. Clin. Lab. Invest.,* Suppl. **68**.

Bosco, C., and Komi, P.V. 1979. Mechanical characteristics and fiber composition of human leg extensor muscles. *Eur. J. Appl. Physiol.* **41**:275-284.

Edstrom, L., and Ekblom, B. 1972. Differences in sizes of red and white muscle fibres in vastus lateralis of musculus quadriceps femoris of normal individuals and athletes. Relation to physical performance. *Scand. J. Clin. Lab. Invest.* **30**:175-181.

Gollnick, P.D., Armstrong, R.B., Saubert, C.W.IV, Piehl, K., and Saltin, B. 1972. Enzyme activity and fiber composition in skeletal muscle of untrained and trained men. *J. Appl. Physiol.* **33**:312-319.

Hulten, B., Thorstensson, A., Sjodin, B., and Karlsson, J. 1975. Relationship between isometric endurance and fiber types in human leg muscles. *Acta Physiol. Scand.* **93**:135-138.

Komi, P.V., and Bosco, C. 1978. Utilization of stored elastic energy in leg extensor muscles by men and women. *Med. Sci. Sports* **10**(4):261-265.

Komi, P.V., Bosco, C., and Pulli, M. 1978. *Muscle elasticity in volleyball players.* Paper presented at the Int. Congress of Biomechanics of Ball Games. Wingate, Israel.

Komi, P.V., and Karlsson, J. 1979. Physical performance, skeletal muscle enzyme activities, and fibre types in monozygous and dizygous twins of both sexes. *Acta Physiol. Scand.,* Suppl. **462**.

Komi, P.V., Klissouras, V., and Karvinen, E. 1973. Genetic variation in neuromuscular performance. *Int. Z. angew. Physiol.* **31**:289-304.

Larsson, L. 1978. Morphological and functional characteristics of the aging skeletal muscle in man. A cross-sectional study. *Acta Physiol. Scand.,* Suppl. **457**.

Margaria, R., Aghemo, P., and Rovelli, E. 1966. Measurement of muscular power (anaerobic) in man. *J. Appl. Physiol.* **21**(5):1661-1664.

Viitasalo, J.T., and Komi, P.V. 1978. Isometric endurance, EMG power spectrum, and fiber composition in human quadriceps muscle. In: E. Asmussen and K. Jorgensen (eds.), *Biomechanics* **VI-A**, pp. 244-250. University Park Press, Baltimore.

The Effects of Glycogen Exhaustion on Maximal Short-term Performance

Ira Jacobs, Peter Kaiser, and **Per Tesch**
Department of Clinical Physiology,
Karolinska Hospital, Stockholm, Sweden

Observed differences in the metabolic and contractile characteristics among skeletal muscle fibers in man have resulted in the distinction of two main types—the slow twitch (ST) and the fast twitch (FT). Speed of muscle contraction and exercise intensity determine which of the two fiber types is predominantly recruited (Burke and Edgerton, 1975). The ST fiber demonstrates a reduced rate of fatigue during repeated contractions when compared to the FT fiber, yet the FT fiber reaches peak tension faster than the ST (Thorstensson, 1976). It was speculated that these differences in contractile features, coupled with known different metabolic profiles (Saltin et al., 1977), might cause the two main fiber types to react differently to glycogen exhaustion.

It has been repeatedly shown that when exercise intensity is 65-85% of $\dot{V}_{O_2}$ max (an intensity that recruits predominantly ST motor units), the depletion of glycogen in the musculature involved seems to be a limiting factor. Exhaustion occurs when extremely low muscle glycogen values are reached (Saltin and Karlsson, 1971). It has previously been demonstrated that prolonged exercise of this intensity results in reduced dynamic strength measurements (Forsberg et al., 1978).

The purpose of this study was to examine the effects of glycogen exhaustion, designed to deplete both main fiber types, on performance of short-term activities such as single maximal contractions and exhaustive, repeated maximal contractions. Significant impairments of performance were observed subsequent to the glycogen depletion program.

Methods

Twelve subjects participated in this study. The group consisted of both athletes (runners) and casual sports participants with a moderate level of physical conditioning.

Strength performance tests were administered according to Thorstensson (1976) on an isokinetic device (Cybex II®, Lumex, New York) before and 1 hr. after a standard exercise program. Briefly, the subjects were required to perform 50 consecutive, maximal extensions of the knee with the lower leg attached to the lever arm of the isokinetic dynamometer. Angular velocity was set to 3.1 rad $\times$ s^{-1}.

Biopsies were obtained from the lateral portion of the thigh (Bergstrom, 1962). Muscle fibers were classified as fast twitch (FT) or slow twitch (ST) after histochemical staining for myofibrillar ATPase (Padykula and Herman, 1955). In addition, six subjects were biopsied following the exercise program to enable histological determinations of qualitative changes in glycogen content of the two main muscle fiber types (Gollnick et al., 1974).

The exercise program consisted of the following activities: running at the maximal velocity that could be maintained for 75 min.; cycling for 30 min. at approximately 70% of $\dot{V}_{O_2}$ max; three bouts of isokinetic, maximal contractions of the quadriceps (one bout = 50 reps at 3.1 rad $\times$ s^{-1}; cycling five times for 1 min. each time at a maximal load. Short periods of rest (15 min.) intervened between different activities.

Results

Maximal strength, expressed as peak torque produced at an angular velocity of 3.1 rad $\times$ s^{-1} was significantly ($p < 0.001$) reduced in all subjects following the exercise program (Figure 1). Based upon the myofibrillar ATPase staining, subjects were divided into two groups: those with greater than 50% FT fiber distribution and those with greater than 50% ST fiber distribution. Both FT and ST groups experienced a significant decrease in peak torque following the exercise program. Prior to the exercise, the FT group demonstrated a higher peak torque value than the ST group, however, this difference was not maintained following the exercise program (Figure 1).

Torque decline, i.e., the absolute difference in Newton meters (Nm) between the peak torque and the average of the 48-50th contraction, was also significantly ($p < 0.05$) reduced after exercise. Mean values were 61 Nm and 51 Nm before and 1 hr. after exercise, respectively. When fiber-type distribution was considered, the FT group demonstrated differences

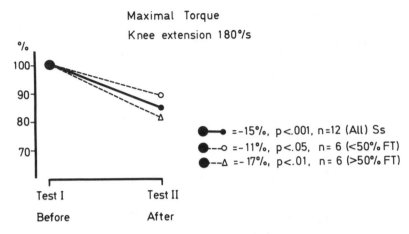

Figure 1—The reduction in maximal torque produced at an angular velocity of 3.1 rad × s^{-1} following glycogen exhaustion.

in torque decline similar to that of the group as a whole; however, this was not evident in the ST group (Figure 2). The FT group also exhibited a greater torque decline than the ST group ($p < 0.05$) prior to exercise, but this difference was not significant following the exercise program.

The histochemical staining for glycogen content revealed that both fiber types were equally depleted following the exercise program. Eighty percent of the ST fibers and 78% of the FT fibers were depleted in the six subjects who were biopsied following the glycogen exhaustion program.

Discussion

The main finding in the present study was the more pronounced decrease in maximal torque production in subjects rich in FT fibers than in subjects rich in ST fibers following glycogen exhaustion.

The task employed to evaluate maximal, short-term performance consisted of isokinetic contractions at a medium angular velocity. Thorstensson (1976) and Coyle et al. (1979) have previously demonstrated that FT fibers are a prerequisite for the maximal muscle contractions at a high speed in man. Forsberg et al. (1978) reported that prolonged exercise (4-8 hr.) reduced maximal torque for dynamic and isometric strength performance characteristics. This reduction was quite pronounced at a relatively slow angular velocity (.5 rad × s^{-1}), but it was apparently not significant at the higher (3.1 rad × s^{-1}) speed. Unfortunately, no data were reported with regard to the fiber type distribution

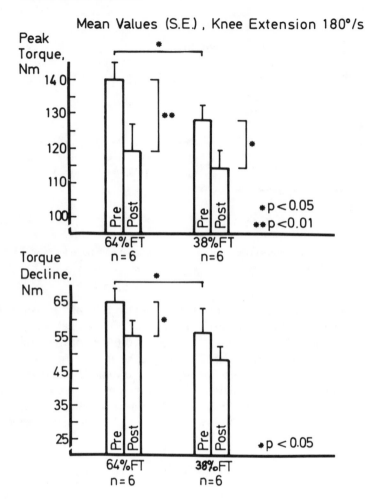

Figure 2—Mean values (S.E.) for peak torque and torque decline before (pre) and after (post) glycogen exhaustion. Subjects are divided into those with a greater and those with less than 50% fast twitch fiber distribution in the vastus lateralis.

of the subjects involved; therefore, its relationship to performance was not discussed. In their study, however, glycogen exhaustion occurred predominantly in the ST fibers, as is evident in the stained sections which we have analyzed from participants in a similar ski race.

Different metabolic profiles are evident when comparing the two main fiber types in human skeletal muscle. The metabolic profile of the ST fiber population favors combustion of free fatty acids (Essen, 1978), whereas that of the FT fiber seems to favor a more pronounced glycogenolytic and carbohydrate combustion metabolism than the ST fibers (Sjodin, 1976). Because the major sources for carbohydrate metabolism in skeletal muscle are the local depots of glycogen, it seems reasonable to suggest that glycogen exhaustion would differentially affect the two fiber types. The ST fiber population may be able to compensate for an impaired carbohydrate availability via a greater utilization of free fatty acids. A similar compensatory mechanism may not be as effective in the FT muscle fibers.

In the present study, both fiber types were equally depleted of their glycogen content. The greater maximal torque and fatigue pattern exhibited by those subjects with a greater FT fiber distribution were not evident 1 hour after the glycogen exhaustion program. One possible interpretation is that a diminished difference exists in terms of contractile characteristics and muscle fatigue development between FT and ST fiber types following glycogen depletion. We assumed that this was due to the concomitant impaired function of the FT muscle fiber. In addition to the direct metabolic effects on the muscle fiber, the possible detrimental effects of fuel shortage on the electromechanical coupling capacity of the contracting fibers must be considered. Such a phenomenon has been suggested by Edwards (1978) as having differential effects on the FT and ST muscle fibers.

Summary

Muscle performance during intense short-term exercise, including single muscular contractions, is impaired by glycogen exhaustion of the musculature involved. The extent of this impairment may be related to FT fiber distribution. The relevancy of these findings is easily applied to many athletic and military endeavors. In soccer players who were biopsied before and after two halves of a normal game, preliminary results have indicated an almost complete emptying of both main fiber types when sections were stained for glycogen content. It is thus quite possible that the explosive contraction required for a single powerful kick of the ball may also be detrimentally affected, in addition to the known reduced endurance performance.

Acknowledgments

The study was supported by grants from the Swedish Medical Research Council (No. 4251), the Research Council of the Swedish Sports Federation, and the Coca-Cola Export Corp., Sweden.

References

Bergstrom, J. 1962. Muscle electrolytes in man. *Scand. J. Clin. Lab. Invest.*, Suppl. **68**.

Burke, R.E., and Edgerton, V.R. 1975. Motor unit properties and selective involvement in movement. In: *Exercise and Sport Sciences Reviews*, Vol. **3**, pp.31-81. Academic Press, NY.

Coyle, E., Costill, D., and Lesmes, G. 1979. Leg extension power and muscle fiber composition. *Med. Sci. Sports* **11**:12-15.

Edwards, R.H.T., Hill, D.K., Jones, D.A., and Merton, P.A. 1977. Fatigue of long duration in human skeletal muscle after exercise. *J. Physiol.* **272**:769-778.

Essen, B. 1978. Studies on the regulation of metabolism in human skeletal muscle using intermittent exercise as an experimental model. *Acta Physiol. Scand.*, Supp. **454**.

Forsberg, A., Tesch, P., and Karlsson, J. 1978. Effects of prolonged exercise on muscle strength performance. In: E. Asmussen and K. Jorgensen (eds.), *Biomechanics* **VI-A**, pp. 62-67, University Park Press, Baltimore.

Gollnick, P.D., Piehl, K., and Saltin, B. 1974. Selective glycogen depletion pattern in human muscle fibers after exercise of varying intensities and at varying pedalling rates. *J. Physiol.* **241**:45-47.

Gydikov, A., and Kosarov, D. 1974. Some features of different motor units in human biceps brachii. *Pflug. Arch.* **347**:75-88.

Padykula, H.A., and Herman, E. 1955. The specificity of the histochemical method of adenosine triphosphatase. *J. Histochem. Cytochem.* **3**:170-195.

Saltin, B., Henriksson, J., Nygaard, E., and Andersen, P. 1977. Fiber types and metabolic potentials of skeletal muscles in sedentary man and endurance runners. *Ann. N.Y. Acad. Sci.* **301**:3-29.

Saltin, B., and Karlsson, J. 1971. Muscle glycogen utilization during work of different intensities. In: B. Pernow and B. Saltin (eds.), *Muscle Metabolism During Exercise*, pp. 289-299. Plenum Press, NY.

Sjodin, B. 1976. Lactate dehydrogenase in human skeletal muscle. *Acta Physiol. Scand.*, Suppl. **436**.

Tesch, P., Sjodin, B., Thorstensson, A., and Karlsson, J. 1978. Muscle fatigue and its relation to lactate accumulation and LDH activity in man. *Acta Physiol. Scand.* **103**:413-420.

Thorstensson, A. 1976. Muscle strength, fiber types and enzyme activities in man. *Acta Physiol. Scand.*, Suppl. **443**.

Muscle Elasticity in Athletes

Carmelo Bosco and **Paavo V. Komi**
University of Jyväskylä, Finland

The intact muscles, as found in the body, consist essentially of two elements—contractile and viscoelastic. These elements were called by Levin and Wyman (1927) "parallel elastic" (PEC) and "series elastic" (SEC) components to indicate that these structures are in parallel or in series, respectively, with the contractile elements in the muscle. During a concentric contraction, the movement begins after the contractile component (CC) has stretched the SEC, which in turn transmits the tension produced by the cross-bridges to the skeletal lever; however, this kind of sequence takes place only seldom in normal human movement. Characteristic to movement is utilization of a stretch-shortening cycle when eccentric (stretch) contraction precedes the concentric (shortening) contraction. This mode of muscular activity is predominant, e.g., in throwing, running, and jumping. The stretch-shortening cycle in these activities implies that the muscles utilize the elastic energy which is stored in them during the prestretch phase (eccentric contraction).

Recently, many investigators have paid attention to the elastic properties of the muscles. For example, Cavagna et al. (1965) have shown that stretching of an activated isolated muscle leads to greater work and power outputs during the shortening phase of contraction. Later, Cavagna and Citterio (1974) concluded that this stretching of an active muscle temporarily modifies its elastic characteristics, which then brings the muscle to work more efficiently during the subsequent positive work (concentric contraction). Thus, it seems that elastic energy is stored during the negative (eccentric) work and recovered in part during the following positive phase. The importance of the elastic energy in human muscular movement has been confirmed in several experiments (Asmussen and Bonde-Petersen, 1974; Cavagna et al., 1971; Komi and Bosco, 1978. In isolated muscle preparations, however, all the nervous connections are cut, and therefore, the improvement noted in the stretching-shortening cycle should be attributed solely to the storage and utilization of elastic energy. On the other hand, in human experiments where the nervous system is intact, part of this "potentiation of performance" through prestretching could be attributed to the reflex potentiation as well (Bosco and Komi, 1979a; Bosco et al., 1981; Schmidtbleicher et al., 1978).

The leg extensor muscles play an important role in many sport activities. It is, therefore, of interest to know what their elastic potential is. This study was undertaken to compare the elastic potential of the leg extensor muscles among athletes of different sport activities. One way to measure this elastic potential of the leg extensor muscles is to test a subject with the test of Komi and Bosco (1978), which is a modification of the techniques introduced by Asmussen and Bonde-Petersen (1974). This consists of maximal voluntary vertical jump on the force-platform with the following different starting positions:

1. From a semisquatting position with no allowance of preparatory counter-movement. This performance is called a jump from a static position (SJ) (90° knee angle). In this condition no appreciable storage and utilization of elastic energy can contribute to the performance. Thus, it can be assumed that the contractile machinery of the leg extensor muscles is primarily responsible for the force production during take-off.

2. From erect standing position on the force-platform, with allowance for counter-movement (CMJ) down to the same position as the starting position in SJ (Figure 1). In this condition, a certain amount of potential elastic energy can be provided to the leg extensor muscles during the eccentric work and utilized at least in part during the following positive work.

3. Dropping on the force-platform from different heights (20-100 cm) with subsequent jumps upwards. This jump is called dropping jump (DJ); and as in the condition of CMJ, potential elastic energy can be stored during the eccentric phase, in which the leg extensor muscles are actively stretched to attenuate the kinetic energy of the body during impact on the platform. The selection of these different jumps assumes that in: (a) SJ, CC is a prime contributor to the performance and (b) the other two jumps, CMJ and DJ, both CC and elastic potentiation contribute to the height jumped. Comparison of performances in SJ to those in CMJ and DJ can, therefore, give information about the elastic characteristics of the leg extensor muscles.

In all test conditions, the subjects kept their hands on their hips during the entire performance. This is necessary to prevent any contribution by the arms, which can be of the order of 10% or more of the total performance (Luhtanen and Komi, 1978). The position of the upper body was also standardized, so that a minimum of flexion and extension of the trunk occurred during the jump.

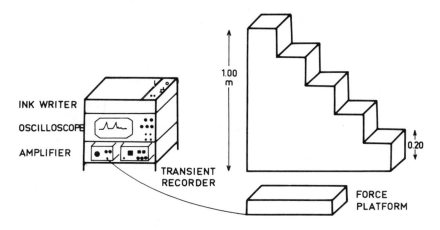

INK WRITER

OSCILLOSCOPE

AMPLIFIER

TRANSIENT
RECORDER

1.00
m

0.20

FORCE
PLATFORM

Figure 1—Schematic representation of instrumentation.

Instrumentation

Figure 1 shows a schematic presentation of the instrumentation used in the study. The force-platform (Komi et al., 1974) recorded the vertical ground reaction force. After the signal was amplified, it was passed through a transient recorder (Transient Store Model 512 A) for immediate display on the oscilloscope and for subsequent tracing on the graphic recorder. Figure 2 is an example of the recorded force-time curves under the different conditions. The stair platform in Figure 1 was used in DJ experiments.

Calculations

By measuring the flight time (t_{air}) from the record (Figure 2), one can calculate the vertical takeoff velocity (V_v) of the center of gravity as follows:

$$V_v = 1/2 \times t_{air} \times g \qquad (1)$$

in which g = acceleration of gravity (9.81 m/s²). The height of rise (h) of the center of gravity can then be computed:

$$h = \frac{V_v^2}{2 \times g} \qquad (2)$$

This method of calculation assumes that the positions of the jumper on the platform were the same in takeoff and in landing. The error of

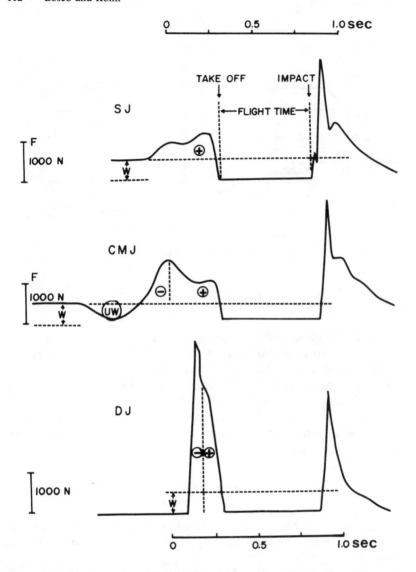

Figure 2—Typical examples of recorded force-time curves under the three different jumping conditions.

measurement, when compared with film analysis has been reported to be of the order of ± 2% (Komi and Bosco, 1978).

The average force ($\overline{F}$) produced during the squatting jump was calculated as follows:

$$\overline{F} = \frac{NI}{t}$$

$$(3)$$

Table 1—Physical Characteristics of the Groups

Groups	N	Age (years)	Weight (kg)	Height (cm)
Students, physical education (S)	16	24.0 ± 1.4	75.4 ± 11.2	176.7 ± 8.3
Runners (800-1,500 m) (R)	13	20.5 ± 3.5	65.7 ± 4.3	179.9 ± 6.4
Shorinij kempo (SK)	8	21.6 ± 3.9	69.9 ± 7.7	176.1 ± 6.0
Soccer players (S$_o$)	6	26.2 ± 5.9	78.5 ± 6.6	183.1 ± 5.1
Volleyball players (VB)	9	24.6 ± 3.3	87.7 ± 6.5	185.8 ± 5.1
Long and triple jumpers (LTJ)	7	23.3 ± 4.5	70.7 ± 3.8	180.1 ± 7.1
High jumpers (HJ)	8	22.6 ± 3.1	81.6 ± 4.8	191.1 ± 4.7
Ski jumpers (SJ)	13	22.3 ± 4.1	70.0 ± 8.2	174.4 ± 6.4

Note. The values indicate the mean ± S.D.

where NI is given by the mass of the subject × V_V and t is the take-off time on the platform.

Subjects

Seventy-eight men participated in the study. They were divided into eight groups as follows: physical education students (16), middle distance runners of national caliber (13), shorinij kempo athletes of national and international level (8), soccer players of international level from Italy (6)[1], volleyball players from the Finnish National Team (9), long and triple jumpers belonging to the Italian National Team (7)[2], high jumpers belonging to the West German, Austrian and Belgian National Teams (8)[2], and ski jumpers from the Finnish National Team (11). Table 1 shows the physical characteristics of the subjects.

Results

When the difference in height of rise of C.G. between CMJ and SJ was

[1]The test was performed in Torino with a force-platform similar to that utilized in our laboratory.

[2]The experiments were performed in Formia (Italian Track and Field College) during an international training camp (Spring 1979), with a force-platform (Kistler type 9261 A). The Sisport-Fiat (Torino-Italy), The Italian Track and Field Association (FIDAL), The Bioengineering Center of Politechnic and The Foundation "Pro Juventude" Milano are gratefully acknowledged for use of their facilities and instruments.

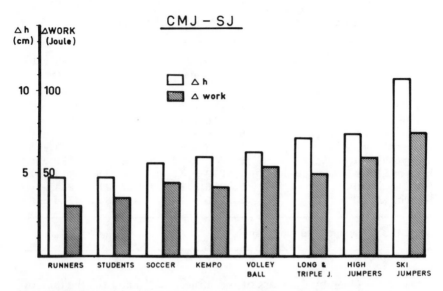

Figure 3—Differences in rise in center of gravity and in work done during countermovement jumping (CMJ) and static jumping (SJ) for selected athletic groups.

compared between the different athlete groups, it was observed that the runners of 800-1,500 m had the least (5 cm) and the ski jumpers had the greatest (8-11 cm) difference. Figure 3 presents this difference also for the other investigated athlete groups. Correspondingly, differences in work (Figure 3) were least (25-35 joules) among the runners and greatest (70-80 joules) among the ski jumpers.

Figure 4 presents the relationship between the height of rise of C.G. in the best drop jump condition and stretch load (dropping height, mgh). As is evident from this figure the runners were able to tolerate and utilize only low stretch loads (300 Nm) as compared to the volleyball players (600 Nm). This optimal stretch load in each group was observed to be related to the average force attained in the squatting jump (Figure 5).

Discussion

From this study, it appears evident that the groups of sportsmen engaged in power events can better utilize the storage of elastic energy during the stretching phase in CMJ. Consequently, the extra work produced in CMJ as compared to SJ also is higher in those groups which trained for explosive power. One might, in addition, speculate that the magnitude of utilization of elastic energy is genetically determined. It has been shown, however, that a special jumping training administered for a period of 18

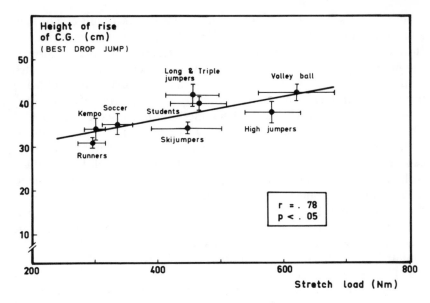

Figure 4—Relationship of rise of C.G. in drop jumping (DJ) and stretch load (Nm) for selected groups of athletes.

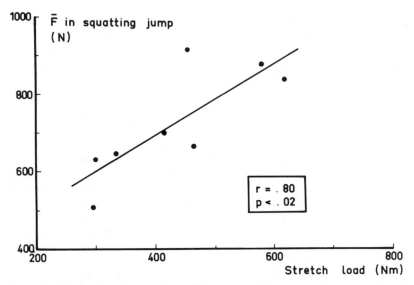

Figure 5—Relationship of mean force (N) attained during squat jumping and optimal stretch load (Nm).

months increased the elastic potential of the leg extensor muscles of long and high jumpers and volleyball players (Bosco et al., 1979a; Komi and Bosco, in preparation). This "bouncing" training not only improved the jumping ability but also increased the tolerance for increased stretch loads. In this connection, the suggestion has been made that bouncing training may influence the contractile and elastic properties of the muscles as well as its proprioceptive feedback mechanism (Bosco et al., 1979b). This would then increase the possibility of storing a greater amount of elastic energy in the muscles without the inhibitory influence of GTO. As can be observed in Figure 4, the groups of athletes which trained daily with eccentric-concentric exercise (stretch-shortening cycle) were able to tolerate high stretching loads and also to obtain higher rises in the C.G. in DJ. On the other hand, the stretching load tolerated by the subject was related to the force produced during SJ. One may speculate that the recruitment pattern of the motor units in leg extensor muscles might be similar in jumping with both conditions. The study of Gillespie et al. (1974) implies that in jumping activities the fast twitch fibers play a primary role in contributing to the performance. This agrees with the finding of a high relationship between percentage of fast twitch fibers and jumping performance (Bosco and Komi, 1979b). Tolerance for high stretch load is important for such an activity as take-off in the long jump. Good long jumpers have demonstrated that they are able to utilize well the elastic potential during the impact phase, where the path of C.G. increases rather than decreases (Bosco et al., 1976). Luhtanen and Komi (1980) reported similar observations by calculating the spring constant values for the leg extensor muscle separately for eccentric and concentric phases. Thus, it can be concluded that in sport activities where stretch-shortening cycle is dominant (e.g., jumping, running, and throwing), the elastic behavior of the muscles plays an important role in influencing the final performance.

References

Asmussen, E., and Bonde-Petersen, F. 1974. Storage of elastic energy in skeletal muscle in man. *Acta Physiol. Scand.* **91**:358-392.

Bosco, C., Ito, A., and Komi, P.V. 1981. Prestretch potentiation of human skeletal muscle during ballistic movement. *Acta Physiol. Scand.* **111**:135-140.

Bosco, C., Luhtanen, P., and Komi, P.V. 1976. Kinetics and kinematics of the take-off in long jump. In: P.V. Komi (ed.), *Biomechanics* **VB**, pp. 174-180. University Park Press, Baltimore.

Bosco, C., Komi, P.V. and Locatelli, E. 1979a. Condiderazioni sull'allenamen to del potenziale elastico del muscolo scheletrico umano. In: *Quadern No. 2 del Centro Studi Coverciano,* 5-18.

Bosco, C., Komi, P.V., and Locatelli, E. 1979b. Physiologische Betrachtungen zum Tiefsprungtraining (Physiological consideration in drop jump training.) *Leistungsport* **6**:434-439.

Cavagna, G.A., and Citterio, G. 1974. Effect of stretching on the elastic characteristics and the contractile component of frog striated muscle. *J. Physiol.* **239**:1-14.

Cavagna, G.A., Komarek, L, Citterio, G., and Margaria, R. 1971. Power output of the previously stretched muscle. In: J. Vredenbregt and J. Wartenweiler (eds.), *Biomechanics II*. Vol. **6**: pp. 159-167. S. Karger, Basel, Switzerland.

Gillespie, C.A., Simpson, D.R., and Edgerton, V.R. 1974. Motor recruitment as reflected by muscle fiber glycogen loss in a prosimian (bushbaby) after running and jumping. *J. Neurol. Neurosurg. Psychiat.* **37**:817-824.

Komi, P.V., and Bosco, C. 1978. Utilization of stored elastic energy in men and women. *Med. Sci. Sports* **10**(4):261-265.

Komi, P.V., Luhtanen, P., and Viljamaa, K. 1974. Measurement of instantaneous contact forces on the force-platform. Research reports from the Department of Biology of Physical Activity 5/74, University of Jyväskylä, Jyväskylä, Finland.

Levin, A., and Wyman, J. 1927. The viscous elastic properties of muscle. *Proc. Roy. Soc. B* **101**:218-243.

Luhtanen, P., and Komi, P.V. 1978. Segmental contribution to forces in vertical jump. *Eur. J. Appl. Physiol.* **38**:181-188.

Luhtanen, P., and Komi, P.V. 1980. Force-, power- and elasticity-velocity relationships in walking, running and jumping. *Eur. J. Appl. Physiol.* **44**:279-289.

Schmidtbleicher, D., Dietz, V., Noth, V., and Antoni, J. 1978. Auftreten und funktionelle Bedeutung des Muskeldehnungsreflexes (Behavior and functional significance of the stretch reflexes of muscles on moderate and fast movements.) *Leistungsport* **6**:480-490.

Medial Lower Leg Pain After Exercise:
A Chronic Compartment Syndrome?

Richard Wallensten
Karolinska Hospital, Stockholm, Sweden

Recurrent pain in the anterior tibial muscle compartment is a well-known phenomenon among athletes (Figure 1). It is produced by exercise and relieved by rest. The chronic form has been well described by several investigators (French and Price, 1962; Mavor, 1956; Leach and Hammond, 1967; Reneman, 1975). It has been shown to be linked to an increased intramuscular pressure in the compartment with muscle ischemia. It is thought that the tight fascial lining of the muscle compartment is too rigid to allow for the swelling of the muscles with exercise, thus creating the increase in pressure.

The more common problem in training and exercise is pain along the anteromedial border of the tibia (Figure 2) corresponding to the deep posterior muscle compartment. The pain is usually localized between the middle and lower third of the tibia and starts with exercise. It is not usually relieved immediately after rest, and can go on for hours and sometimes even days. It has been suggested that this is also a compartment syndrome (D'Ambrosia et al., 1977; Puranen, 1974; Snook, 1975). The basis for this suggestion has been the nature of the symptoms and the fact that they are relieved by surgical release of the fascia from the tibia at the site of pain.

In order to find out whether the so-called shin splint or medial lower leg pain after exercise is a chronic compartment syndrome, athletes with lower leg pain were examined for intramuscular pressure, muscle fiber distribution, and metabolism before and after fasciotomy.

Methods

We examined three subjects with pain in the anterior tibial compart-

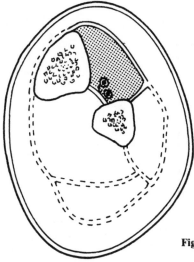

Figure 1—The anterior tibial muscle compartment.

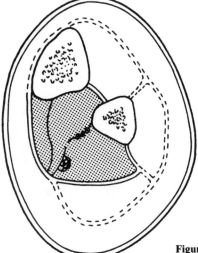

Figure 2—The deep posterior muscle compartment.

ment, five with pain in the deep posterior compartment, and as controls, five healthy volunteers. In addition, participants in an 85 km cross-country ski race and a city marathon race were examined.

Intramuscular pressure was recorded with the wick method (Mubarak et al., 1976) before and after exercise, consisting of footwork using an isokinetic dynamometer. Needle biopsies (Bergstrom, 1962) from the muscles in the compartments were analyzed in terms of fiber distribution, water, and lactate content. The symptomatic subjects were also ex-

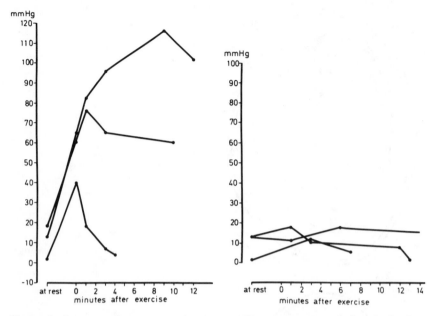

Figure 3—Intramuscular pressure in the anterior compartment before and after fasciotomy.

amined several months after fasciotomy of the afflicted compartment.

Results

Intramuscular pressure was much elevated in the subjects with pain in the anterior tibial compartment (Figure 3) in comparison with the volunteers after exercise (Figure 4). They also took a longer time to reach the pre-exercise resting level.

In subjects with pain on the medial side of the tibia, pressure was never elevated above normal values even after heavy exercise forced the individual to stop because of pain (Figure 5). They did not differ from the control subjects.

After fasciotomy, pressure in the anterior tibial compartment was normalized and did not increase after exercise (Figure 3). Water content in the muscles was around 75%. There was no difference between the different groups of subjects before or after exercise.

Fiber typing into slow and fast twitch fibers showed a predominance of slow twitch fibers in both compartments in all subjects. Because most of the individuals examined trained for middle or long distance running, this was to be expected.

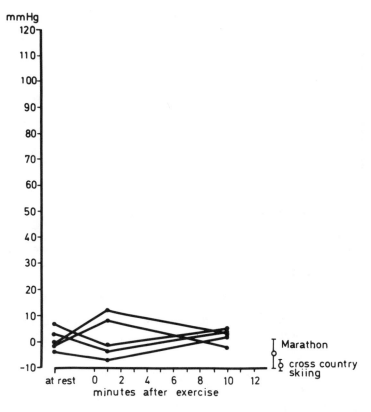

Figure 4—Intramuscular pressure in the anterior compartment in healthy subjects.

The muscle lactate determinations showed that, in subjects with anterior tibial pain, exercising the leg raised muscle lactate to abnormally high levels (Figure 6). After the operation, the same increase did not occur. The subjects with medial pain (Figure 6) and the volunteers (Fig. 7) did not increase muscle lactate after exercise in the same way.

Discussion

The results show that pain in the anterior tibial compartment after exercise is accompanied by a rise in intramuscular pressure to a level where it exceeds the capillary blood pressure and an ischemic situation occurs. This is reflected in the rise of lactate indicating an anaerobic metabolism. Fasciotomy relieves this. In subjects with medial pain, none of these changes occurred, either after exercise or fasciotomy. Though they were relieved from pain by the operation, there was no evidence of ischemia

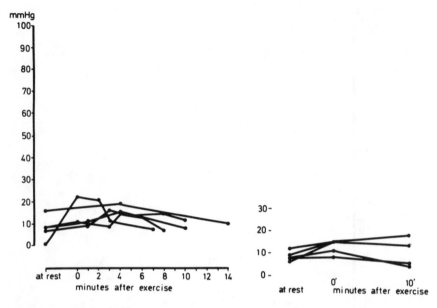

Figure 5—Intramuscular pressure in the deep posterior compartment in patients with medial pain and healthy subjects.

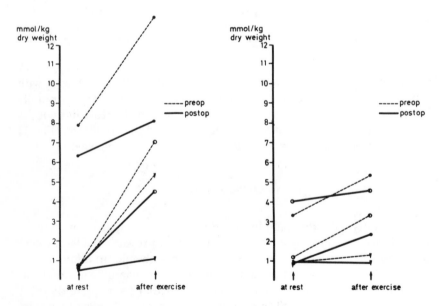

Figure 6—Muscle lactate in patients with pain in the anterior or deep posterior compartment.

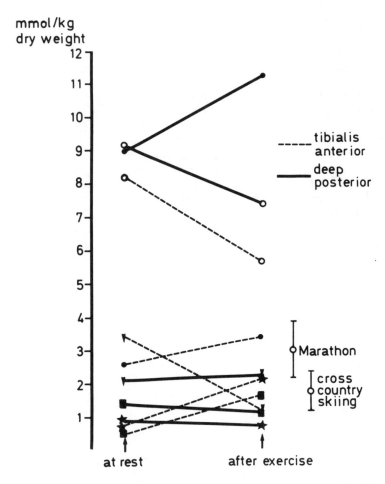

Figure 7—Muscle lactate in the anterior and deep posterior compartments in healthy subjects.

and the symptoms could, therefore, not be defined as a chronic compartment syndrome as Puranen suggested (1974). It may be an overuse inflammation or a mechanical problem at the insertion on the tibia where the fascia meets the periosteal tissue, which is very sensitive to pain. This, however, requires further study.

References

D'Ambrosia, R.D., Zelis, R.F., Chuinard, R.G., and Wilmore, J. 1977. Interstitial pressure measurements in the anterior and posterior compartments in

124   Wallensten

athletes with shin splints. *Am. J. Sports Med.* **5**:127-131.

Bergstrom, J. 1962. Muscle electrolytes in man. *Scand. J. Clin. Lab. Invest.*, Suppl. **68**.

French, E.B., and Price, W.H. 1962. Anterior tibial pain. *Brit. Med. J.* **2**:1290-1296.

Leach, R.E., Hammond, G., and Stryker, W. 1967. Anterior tibial compartment syndrome. Acute and chronic. *J. Bone Jt. Surg.* **49 A**: 451-462.

Mavor, G.E. 1956. The anterior tibial syndrome. *J. Bone Jt. Surg.* **38 B**: 513-517.

Mubarak, S.J., Hargens, A.R., Owen, C.A., Garetto, L.P., and Akeson, W.H. 1976. The wick catheter technique for measurement of intramuscular pressure. A new research and clinical tool. *J. Bone Jt. Surg.* **58 A**:1016-1020.

Puranen, J. 1974. The medial tibial syndrome. Exercise ischemia in the medial fascial compartment of the leg. *J. Bone Jt. Surg.* **56 B**: 712-715.

Reneman, R.S. 1975. The anterior and the lateral compartmental syndrome of the leg due to intensive use of muscles. *Clin. Orthop. Related Res.* **113**:69-79.

Snook, G.A. 1975. Intermittent claudication in athletes. *J. Sports Med.* **3**:71-75.

Exercise Under Different Environmental Conditions

The Child Athlete and Thermoregulation

Oded Bar-Or
Wingate Institute for Physical Education and Sport, Israel

Optimal climatic conditions have long been recognized as essential when athletic performance is to be maximized. Suboptimal climates, in which the environment is too hot, too humid, or too cold, have a detrimental effect on performance and may jeopardize the health of the athlete.

Concepts such as acclimitization to heat, fluid replacement, evaporative cooling, solar radiation, and heat intolerance are becoming part and parcel of modern coaching strategy. Most knowledge in this field is related to the adult athlete. Recent years have witnessed a continuous rise in the number of children who are exposed to highly intense training regimens. It is therefore important to know whether the child athlete reacts the same way as an adult to climatic stress. Such information is of further relevance because young children are more prone than adults to heat-related diseases, as is suggested by epidemiologic evidence.

It is the aim of this article to review data on thermoregulation of the child and preadolescent athlete. Emphasis will be given to those aspects in which the child responds *differently* from the adult and to implications for coaching and health supervision.

Theoretical Considerations

Certain morphological and functional differences between children and adults have a bearing on thermoregulatory efficiency. These are listed in Table 1.

The main age-related geometric difference is the greater surface area per unit body mass of children. A 7-year-old child has some 35-40% more surface per kg body weight than a young adult. This implies a greater heat transfer between the skin of the child and the environment,

Table 1—Main Morphological and Functional Differences Between Children and Adults and Their Implications for Thermoregulation

Typical of children	Effect on thermoregulation
Greater surface area/mass ratio	Greater rates of heat exchange skin-environment
Greater energy expenditure during walking and running	Greater production of metabolic heat per kg body weight
Lower sweating rate at rest and exercise	Potentially lower capacity for evaporative cooling
Lower cardiac output at a given metabolic level	Lower capacity for heat convection from body core to periphery

through conduction, convection, and radiation. Such heat transfer is especially great in climatic extremes when ambient temperature (T_{amb}) is much higher or much lower than skin temperature (T_{sk}). The child will, therefore, be at a distinct disadvantage when exposed to such climatic extremes.

When a child and an adult walk or run side by side, energy expenditure per kg body weight is higher for the child. Differences can be as high as 20-30%, whether in neutral (Astrand, 1952) or in hot (Bar-Or et al., 1969, cf. Haymes et al., 1974) climates. The end result is that children produce more metabolic heat for an equal task. This may be a distinct disadvantage in strenuous athletic activities, especially when climatic heat stress is superimposed. The reason for age-related differences in energy expenditure is currently being studied in our laboratory by cinematography and metabolic evaluation.

Especially among males, the sweating rate in the exercising child is lower than in adults, whether calculated in absolute values or per unit area of skin (Drinkwater et al., 1977; Haymes et al., 1975; Inbar, 1978; Sohar and Shapira, 1965; Van Beaumont, 1965; Wagner et al., 1972). The reason is not a smaller population density of glands of the child but rather a smaller production per gland (Bar-Or, 1980). Although reduced sweating capacity is conceptually a handicap for children, one cannot rule out the possibility that the child evaporates sweat more efficiently. Evaporation from many small drops may be more economical than evaporation from larger drops spread further apart; however, no information is available regarding this hypothesis.

For a given metabolic level the cardiac output of children is somewhat lower than that of adults, both in neutral environments (Bar-Or et al., 1971; Eriksson, 1971) and in hot climates (Drinkwater et al., 1977). Assuming that skin blood flow during strenuous activity may be limited by the available cardiac output, convective heat loss from body core to the skin is potentially deficient in children.

In conclusion, theoretical considerations suggest that the thermoregulatory capacity of children may be deficient when compared with adults, especially during exposure to climatic extremes. The following is a brief discussion of data specifically relevant to the child athlete who is exposed to hot or cold climates.

Acclimatization to Exercise in the Heat

Acclimatization to heat is an important process for any athlete who has to travel from cool to warmer climates and is expected to perform well. It is also of relevance at the onset of a climatic heat wave. A non-acclimatized athlete who exerts on a hot day will not perform well and his health may be jeopardized. Inbar (1978) and Wagner et al. (1972) found that children and preadolescents can acclimatize to exercise in the heat, but to a lesser degree than adults. The *rate* of acclimatization is lower in children, such that they need more exposures until the objective benefit is manifested. On the other hand, their subjective well-being, as determined by exercise perception, develops faster than in adults (Bar-Or, 1980; Bar-Or and Inbar, 1977). Such a discrepancy may instill in the child a false sense of confidence. He or she may be less inhibited and thus overexert in hot weather. Coaches and team physicians should be aware of this phenomenon and curtail training of the nonacclimatized child during the first 2 to 3 days of a sudden rise in climatic heat stress.

Omission on their part to enforce such precautions may involve a great risk to the child. Only a few epidemiologic studies are available on the acclimatization status of young athletes who were victims of heat stroke. One common denominator for heat stroke fatalities among high school American football players is the early stage of the season in which the event occurred. The great majority of the victims sustained heat stroke on the first or second day of practice when in all probability they were not yet acclimatized (Barcenas et al., 1976; Fox et al., 1966; Redfearn and Murphy, 1969).

Heat Tolerance of Children

When exercising in a neutral or moderately warm environment, children thermoregulate as efficiently as young adults (Bar-Or, 1980; Drinkwater et al., 1977; Gullestad, 1975; Haymes et al., 1974; Inbar, 1978). On the other hand, when air temperature reaches 45 ° C or more, the exercising child is at a distinct disadvantage (Bar-Or, 1980; Dill et al.,

1966; Drinkwater and Horvath, 1979; Drinkwater et al., 1977; Haymes et al., 1974; Wagner et al., 1972). Effective temperature which exceeds 30° was found intolerable to children exercising at moderate intensities (40-50% of aerobic capacity). One reason for such intolerance is the large surface area/mass ratio which enhances heat flow from the environment. Such flow is especially amplified when the T_{amb}-T_{sk} gradient is high. Another suggested cause (Drinkwater et al., 1977) is the relatively low central blood volume and blood flow to the central organs of children walking in the heat.

The practical implication is to protect the child athlete from overexerting while exposed to extremely hot climates, especially when his task requires activity of 30 min. or more. No information is available on the ability of children exposed to heat to sustain high intensity exercise lasting only a few minutes. For supramaximal activities of less than 1 min., however, neither heat nor high humidity proved detrimental to children (Dotan and Bar-Or, in preparation).

Dehydration

The relationship between dehydration and athletic activity is two-faceted: on the one hand, the inadvertent fluid loss which is not replenished by sufficient intake (e.g., in a marathon race), and on the other, the deliberate fluid deficit advocated by coaches and athletes in sports such as wrestling, judo, or boxing.

Whatever the cause, dehydration may be detrimental to physiological and mental functions which are relevant to athletic performance and to the well-being of the athlete. Ample evidence indicates that the dehydrated child is more prone to heat-related illness than is the fully hydrated one (e.g., Danks et al., 1962; Taj-Eldin and Falaki, 1968). Yet, only a little information is available to compare the effects of dehydration on exercising children and adults. In a recent study from our laboratory (Bar-Or et al., 1980), 10- to 12-year-old boys were found to voluntarily dehydrate while intermittently exercising (45% $\dot{V}_{O_2}$ max) for 3.5 hr. in a hot climate (39°C, 45% relative humidity). The rate of fluid loss was similar to that described for adults who performed similar tasks. One difference, though, was that, for a given percentage of weight loss, the children had a distinctly greater rise in core temperature.

The above protocol induced only mild levels of dehydration (up to 2% of initial body weight). No data are available which systematically compare the response of exercising children and adults to higher degrees of dehydration; however, for the sake of safety, one should assume that the child athlete is at least as adversely affected by dehydration as are adults.

This topic is especially relevant to wrestling, which is a popular high school (and in some countries, elementary school) sport. In a survey among high school wrestlers (Tipton and Tcheng, 1970), weight losses as high as 15% were induced during a 10-day period prior to weighing-in. The youngest and smallest wrestlers lost relatively more than the older ones. Assuming that much of this weight loss reflected fluid deficit, these children exposed themselves to extremely high levels of dehydration. In a recent study (Allen et al., 1977), high school wrestlers who dehydrated up to 4.6% of initial body weight were found to lose nearly 5% of their plasma volume. It is conceivable that, in addition to a decrement in hemodynamic function, such athletes may also have thermoregulatory deficiency.

It is often the decision of the coach as to whether and how much a young athlete should deliberately dehydrate. Until proven otherwise, induced dehydration among children should be considered a health hazard, with potential long-term consequences to growth. This approach has been adopted by the American College of Sports Medicine, which recently issued a Position Stand on weight loss in wrestling (American College of Sports Medicine, 1976).

Exercise in Cold Environments

Exposure to the cold may induce local cooling and injury to exposed skin, as well as heat loss from the entire body. Local cooling may take place both at rest and during exercise. It can easily be prevented by proper clothing. Generalized heat loss may pose a serious problem at rest but generally not during intense exercise, where metabolic heat production more than compensates for the heat loss via the skin. Aquatic sports are an exception. Due to the high thermal conductivity of water (25 times that of air), heat transfer from skin to water in a swimmer may be as high as 30 times that in a person exercising on land (Buskirk, 1978).

Since the rate of heat conduction from skin to water depends on the contact area between the two media, a swimming child who has a relatively larger surface area should lose more heat per kg body weight than a swimming adult. Indeed, when 8- to 19-year-old trained swimmers were exposed to 20.3 °C (swimming at four to five times their resting metabolic rate), the younger ones had a distinctly shorter endurance time and their core temperature dropped 2-3 °C within some 20 min. The older swimmers had a 50-60% longer endurance time and their core temperature dropped only marginally (Sloan and Keatinge, 1973). The main reasons for such a difference were the lower thickness of subcutaneous fat and the relatively larger surface area in the young children. The cooler the water, the more obvious the age-related difference. Coaches who train their athletes in cool water should be aware of this phenomenon, especially when working with small, lean individuals.

Summary

Our current knowledge of the thermoregulatory characteristics of exercising children includes the following:

1. Children have limited tolerance time in hot climates.
2. They generally produce less sweat than young adults.
3. They can acclimatize to heat but may require more exposures than adults.
4. They will voluntarily dehydrate.
5. Dehydration in exercising children may lead to a greater thermal load than among young adults.
6. Young children are more susceptible than young adults to heat-related illness.
7. When exposed to the cold, children will lose greater amounts of heat.

The information presented in this paper is based on fragmentary evidence. Valid interpretation of comparative data is sometimes difficult, because metabolic loads and climatic heat stress are not properly equated across ages (see Drinkwater and Horvath, 1979). In addition, ethical considerations preclude the use with children of research techniques commonly used with adults. This may slow down any further accumulation of information.

Topics to be studied in the future include:

1. What is the *implication* of the reduced sweating capacity of the child?
2. What are the physiological, performance and health consequences of high levels of dehydration in the exercising child?
3. What are the sex differences in thermoregulation of children and are they dependent on level of maturation?
4. What are the combined effects of exercise and climate on the ambulatory sick child?

Acknowledgments

The author is indebted to Ms. Dinah Figenbaum for her devotion and help in preparing this manuscript.

The original data in this review are from studies supported by the Sports and

Physical Education Authority, Ministry of Education and Culture, Israel. Most of these studies were done with Omri Inbar and Raffy Dotan.

References

Allen, T.E., Smith, D.P., and Killer, D.K. 1977. Hemodynamic response to submaximal exercise after dehydration and rehydration in high school wrestlers. *Med. Sci. Sports* **9**:159-163.

American College of Sports Medicine. 1976. Position stand on weight loss in wrestlers. *Med. Sci. Sports* **8**(2): XI-XIII.

Astrand, P.O. 1952. Experimental studies of physical working capacity in relation to sex and age. Munksgaard, Copenhagen.

Barcenas, C., Hoeffler, H.P., and Lie, J.T. 1976. Obesity, football, dog days and siriasis: A deadly combination. *Am. Heart J.* **92**:237-244.

Bar-Or, O. 1980. Climate and the exercising child—A review. *Int. J. Sports Med.* **1**:53-65.

Bar-Or, O., Dotan, R., Inbar, O., Rothstein, A., and Zonder, H. 1980. Voluntary hypohydration in 10- to 12-year-old boys. *J. Appl. Physiol. Respirat. Environ. Ex. Physiol.* **48**:104-108.

Bar-Or.,O., and Inbar,O. 1977. Relationship between perceptual and physiological changes during heat acclimatization in 8- to 10-year old boys. In: H. Lavalee and R.J. Shephard (eds.), *Frontier of Activity and Child Health*, pp. 205-214.

Bar-Or, O., Lundegren, H.M., and Buskirk, E.R. 1969. Heat tolerance of exercising lean and obese women. *J. Appl. Physiol.* **26**:403-409.

Bar-Or, O., Shephard, R.J., and Allen, C.L. 1971. Cardiac output of 10- to 13-year-old boys and girls during submaximal exercise. *J. Appl. Physiol.* **30**:219-233.

Buskirk, E.R. 1978. Cold stress: A selective review. In: L.J. Folinsbee, (eds.), *Environmental Stress—Individual Human Adaptations*, pp. 249-266. Academic Press, New York, NY.

Danks, D.M., Webb, D.W., and Allen, J. 1962. Heat illness in infants and young children: A study of 47 cases. *Br. Med. J.* **5300**:8P-9P.

Dill, D.B., Hall, F.G., and Van Beaumont, W. 1966. Sweat chloride concentration, sweat rate; metabolic rate, skin temperature and age. *J. Appl. Physiol.* **21**:99-106.

Drinkwater, B.L., and Horvath, S.M. 1979. Heat tolerance and aging. *Med. Sci. Sports* **11**:49-55.

Drinkwater, B.L., Kupprat, I.C., Denton, J.E., Crist, J.L., and Horvath, S.M. 1977. Response of prepubertal girls and college women to work in the heat. *J. Appl. Physiol.* **43**:1046-1053.

Eriksson, B.O. 1971. Cardiac output during exercise in pubertal boys. *Acta Paed. Scand.*, Suppl. **217**:53-55.

Fox, E.L., Mathews, D.K., Kaufman, W.S., and Bowers, R.W. 1966. Effects of football equipment on thermal balance and energy cost during exercise. *Res. Q. Am. Assoc. Health Phys. Ed.* **37**:332-339.

Gullestad, R. 1975. Temperature regulation in children during exercise. *Acta Pediatr. Scand.* **64**:257-263.

Haymes, E.M., Buskirk, E.R., Hodgson, J.L., Lundegren, H.M., and Nicholas, W.C. 1974. Heat tolerance of exercising lean and heavy prepubertal girls. *J. Appl. Physiol.* **36**:566-571, 1974.

Haymes, E.M., McCormick, R.J., and Buskirk, E.R. 1975. Heat tolerance of exercising lean and obese boys. *J. Appl. Physiol.* **39**:257-461.

Inbar, Omri. 1978. *Acclimatization to Dry and Hot Environment in Young Adults and in Children 8-10 Years Old.* Ph.D. dissertation, Columbia University, New York, NY.

Redfearn, J.A.Jr., and Murphy, R.J. 1969. History of heat stroke in a football trainee. *J. Am. Med. Assoc.* **208**:699-700.

Sloan, R.E.G., and Keatinge, W.R. 1973. Cooling rates of young people swimming in cold water. *J. Appl. Physiol.* **35**:371-375.

Sohar, E., and Shapira, Y. 1965. The physiological reactions of women and children marching during heat (abstract). *Proc. Isr. Physiol. Pharmacol. Soc.* **1**:50.

Taj-Eldin, S., and Falaki, N. 1968. Heat illness in infants and small children in desert climates. *J. Trop. Med. Hyg.* **71**:100-104.

Tipton, C.M., and Tcheng, T. 1970. Iowa wrestling study. Weight loss in high school students. *J. Am. Med. Assoc.* **214**:1269-1274.

Van Beaumont, W. 1965. Thermoregulation in desert heat with respect to age (abstract). *Physiologist* **8**:294.

Wagner, J.A., Robinson, S., Tzankoff, S.P., and Marino, R.P. 1972. Heat tolerance and acclimatization to work in the heat in relation to age. *J. Appl. Physiol.* **33**:616-622.

Ultrastructural Changes in Myocardial Cells Under Conditions of High Altitude Training

H.-J. Appell and **C. Stang-Voss**
Institute of Experimental Morphology,
Deutsche Sporthochschule, Köln, Germany

High altitude training has been employed since the Olympics in Mexico City, and the possible effects of physical performance under hypoxic conditions are still being disputed today. Considering recent records in mountaineering and even in high altitude skiing as a popular sport, one is faced with the problem of the pathogenic risk of exercising under hypoxic conditions. It is known that functional disturbances progress with increasing altitude (Ruff and Strughold, 1957; Van Liere and Stickney, 1963). The liver and the heart are most susceptible as revealed in the extensive studies of Franz Buchner in the thirties and forties of this century (Grundmann, 1975). For example, right ventricular hypertrophy in the heart occurs as a result of hypoxic pulmonary hypertension (Caspari et al., 1978). According to Eppinger's (1931) theory of "hypoxia-induced insufficiency of the hypertrophied heart," the myocardium will be supplied with less oxygen due to the growing diameters of the myocytes (Frank, 1950), which finally leads to heart insufficiency. In the athlete's heart, however, the simultaneous and uniform hypertrophy of both ventricles, induced by physical training, is compensated by an appropriate capillary supply under normal circumstances.

In the present study, both of these hypertrophy-stimulating effects will be combined, the one (hypoxia) affecting only the right ventricle. The specific purpose was to examine the adaptive capacity of myocardium to increased loads under hypoxic conditions similar to those occurring in high altitude training. It is open to question whether the compensated state of the athlete's heart will lose its balance in an hypoxic environment, leading to chronic heart insufficiency.

As experimental model, Japanese waltzing mice were used, which have a genetically determined motor activity due to an inborn defect of the inner ear (Gruneberg, 1952). Exposing these mice to hypobaric pressures, i.e., simulated altitude, was regarded as similar to the conditions an athlete experiences in training at high altitude.

Materials and Methods

Twenty young but full-grown male Japanese waltzing mice (*Mus wagneri rotans*) were subdivided into three groups and were held in a low pressure chamber at 525 Torr (approx. 3,000 m altitude) for 7, 14, and 21 days, respectively. The animals were then sacrificed and portions of the right ventricular myocardium were removed. The sample was prepared for electron microscopy (EM) as follows: fixation in 2.5% glutaraldehyde in 0.1 m Na-cacodylate buffer and 1% OsO_4 in the same buffer; dehydration in graded alcohol; contrasting "en bloc" with 1% uranylacetate and 0.5% phosphotungstic acid, embedding in Epon 812; and ultrathin sections on a LKB III Ultrotome. All EM-investigations were carried out on a ZEISS EM 10.

Results

After 7 days of hypoxia, the most conspicuous alterations of the myocardiocytes appeared in the mitochondria (Figure 1), which were swollen and their matrix was light and structureless. In addition, there were signs of cristolysis. This degenerative process was reversible, as was revealed by the formation of new, mainly small, mitochondria after 14 days. At this point, further changes occurred in the contractile material, due to hypertrophy (Figure 2). In most cases, there were light areas in the cells containing thick and thin filaments which showed either no arrangement at all or were oriented parallel, without forming sarcomeres. These bundles were attached to the sarcolemma to form distinct myofibrils. Abundant free ribosomes and well-developed Golgi cisternae were visible (Figure 3), supporting the progressive process of hypertrophy. On the other hand, there was a marked appearance of lipofuscine after 14 days (Figure 3), which was primarily deposited adjacent to the sarcolemma or around the nucleus. The origin of lipofuscine may possibly be derived from vacuoles containing destroyed mitochondria or amorphous electron-dense material. Occasionally, there were myotube-like cells (Figure 4) with a light cytoplasm containing endoplasmic reticulum and free ribosomes as well as thin filaments which were attached at various points to the Z-disc material. After 21 days of hypoxia, many myocytes showed peculiar signs of beginning necrosis (Figure 5), the sarcomeres

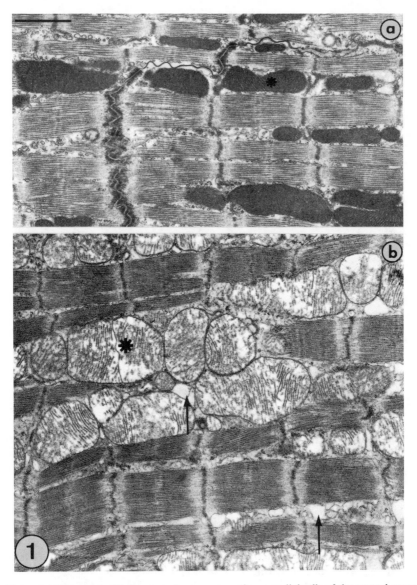

Figure 1—Compared with the normal appearance of myocardial cells of the control group (a), the mitochondria (asterisk) are swollen after 7 days of hypoxia (b), and the sarcoplasmic reticulum is distended (arrow). The bar represents 1 micron (in all figures).

were totally destroyed or myolytically changed, containing aberrant filaments, and the whole cell seemed to be disorganized in a spectacular manner.

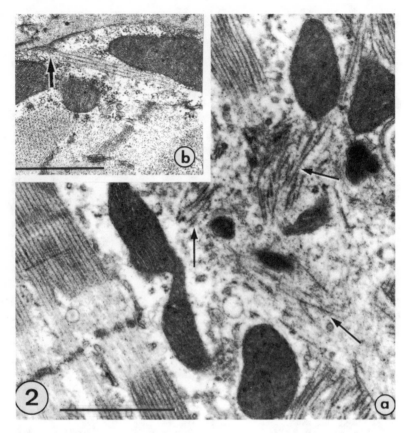

Figure 2—a) During progressive hypertrophy, clusters of thick and thin filaments appear, which are partly associated to small bundles (arrow). 7 days of hypoxia. b) A bundle of filaments is inserted at a dense zone of the sarcolemma (arrow). 14 days hypoxia.

Discussion

The changes occurring in the myocardium during exposure to hypoxia were not that stringently dependent upon time, and they will therefore be discussed with regard to the structural elements.

Mitochondrial alterations in the myocardium as seen after 7 days hypoxia are described under experimental conditions of acute hypoxia to the tissue (Ferrans and Roberts, 1971), e.g., blood-letting or aortic stenosis (Buchner and Onishi, 1970; Hatt and Swynghedauw, 1968; Novi, 1968), as well as after prolonged exhaustive exercise (Paniagua et al., 1977), which are both conditions of extreme stress to the myocytes. The conditions designed in the present experiment (hypoxia and motor activity) are moderate when they are separated, but they seem to be

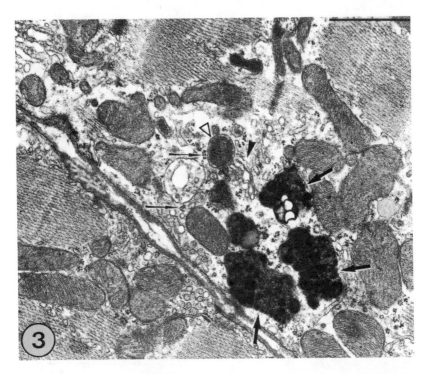

Figure 3—After 14 days of hypoxia, lipofuscine deposits (arrow) are visible as well as vacuoles containing dense material (open arrow); furthermore, there are abundant ribosomes (small arrow) and Golgi cisternae (arrowhead).

cumulative in their effect when combined. The severe initial damage does not quite lead to necroses but is altered by regenerative processes as new mitochondria are formed. Moreover, during the development of hypertrophy, new filaments are built up which are associated with regular fibrils arising from dense zones of the sarcolemma. This pattern is characteristic during hypertrophy (Eriskovskaya and Cellarius, 1977; Hatt et al., 1979) and could lead to fibrillar organizations which arise from contraction insufficiency because of a missing parallelism of the fibrils (Imamura, 1978). Other structural peculiarities of the contractile material which have been reported to occur after hypoxia or exhaustive exercise in the Z-disc (Goldstein et al., 1977) or the sarcomeric pattern (Paniagua et al., 1977) could not be observed and are thought to be artificially caused (Chase et al., 1978). It is assumed that hypertrophy occurs in the myocardium and that the ventricular mass increases because of hyperplasia (Hatt et al., 1979), which is supported by autoradiographic studies (Wachtlova et al., 1977). Even in the myocardium, new myocytes have been formed by myoblasts (Legato, 1972), although myo-

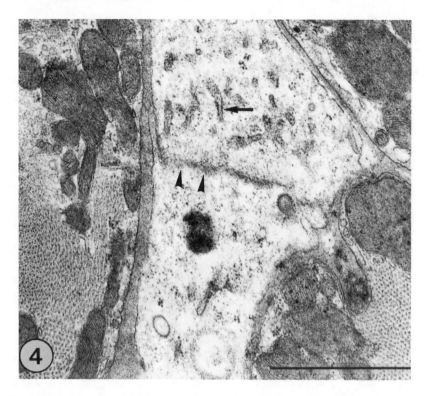

Figure 4—A light cell, probably a myotube, contains tubular elements due to endoplasmic reticulum (arrow) and free ribosomes; thin filaments seem to become attached to Z-disc-like dense material (arrowhead). 14 days of hypoxia.

tubes are not assumed to play as important a role in myocardial regeneration as in skeletal muscle (Hudgson and Field, 1973).

In contrast to these progressive changes, the abundance of lipofuscine from the fourteenth day of hypoxia is apparently due to a destructive process. This has never been described under similar experimental conditions, but analogous changes occur during acute myocardial anoxia (Laufer, 1971). The formation of lipofuscine is interpreted as a wasting of the myocytes due to aging and termed "brown atrophy." The destruction of cells is further supported by myolytic signs. It can therefore be assumed that the progressive changes due to hypertrophy are not sufficiently comparable to those caused by exercise stress at high altitude; hence, the myocytes become insufficient, producing lipofuscine as a sign of premature aging of the heart. Sedentary animals showed no degenerative changes under the same hypoxic conditions. Thus, it can be assumed that the right ventricular myocytes are able to adapt to hypoxia both by means of hypertrophy and through their capillary supply (Turek

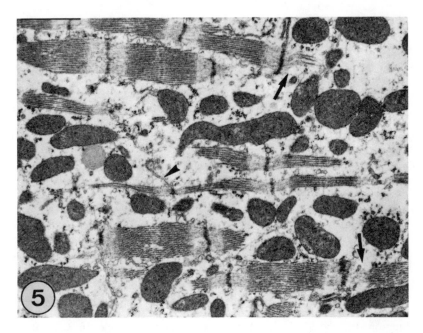

Figure 5—After 21 days of hypoxia, signs of myocardial insufficiency are visible: the myofibrils are myolytically changed (arrow), which is accompanied by the appearance of aberrant filaments (arrowhead).

et al., 1972), but only when the stress is not exaggerated by additional motor activity. Although conclusions derived from animal experiments should not be transferred to man without reservations, these results suggest that high altitude training without previous adaptation to the hypoxic environment could lead to myocardial injury.

References

Buchner, F., and Onishi, S. 1970. *Herzhypertrophie und Herzinsuffizienz in der Sicht der Elektronenmikroskopie.* (Heart Hypertrophy and Insufficiency in Electron Microscopy.) Urban and Schwarzenberg, Munich-Berlin-Vienna.

Caspari, P.G., Newcomb, M., Gibson, K., and Harris, P. 1978. Myocardial collagen, the effects of right ventricular hypertrophy and its involution induced by changes in atmospheric pressure. *Cardiovasc. Res.* **12**:173-178.

Chase, D., Dasse, K., Goldberg, A.H., and Ullrich, W.C. 1978. Influence of acute hypoxia on Z-line width of cardiac muscle. *J. Mol. Cell. Cardiol.* **10**:1077-1080.

Eppinger, H. 1931. Zur Pathologie der Kreislaufregulationen. (Pathology of circulation regulation.) *Hdb. norm. path. Physiol.* **16/2**:1289-1412, Berlin.

Eriskovskaya, N.K., and Cellarius, Y.G. 1977. Formation of transversely oriented myofibrils in the cardiomyocytes in cardiac hypertrophy. *Bull. Ex.*

Biol. **83**:895-898.

Ferrans, V.J., and Roberts, W.C. 1971. Myocardial ultrastructure in acute and chronic hypoxia. *Cardiology* **56**:144-160.

Frank, A. 1950. Experimentelle Herzhypertrophie. (Experimental heart hypertrophy.) *Z. ges. exp. Med.* **115**:312-339.

Goldstein, M.A., Thyrum, P.T., Murphy, D.L., Martin, J.H., and Schwartz, A. 1977. Ultrastructural and contractile characteristics of isolated papillary muscle exposed to acute hypoxia. *J. Mol. Cell. Cardiol.* **9**:285-295.

Gruneberg, H. 1952. *The Genetics of the Mouse*, pp. 78-104. Martinus Nijhoff, Netherlands.

Grundmann, E. (ed.). 1975. Franz Buchner: Hypoxie, Beitrage aus den Jahren 1932-1972. (Franz Buchner: Hypoxia, contributions from 1932-1972.) Springer, Berlin-Heidelberg-New York.

Hatt, P.Y., Jouannot, P., and Moravec, J. 1979. Le ventricle gauche aux differentes etapes d'une double surcharge mechanique. Etude au microscope electronique chez le rat. (The left ventricle at different stages in two-step mechanical overloading. Electron microscopic study in the rat.) *Path. Biol.* **27**:67-77.

Hatt, P.Y., and Swynghedauw, B. 1968. Electron microscopic study of myocardium in experimental heart insufficiency. In: R. Reindell (ed.), *Herzinsuffizienz. Pathophysiologie und Klinik*. Stuttgart.

Hudgson, P., and Field, E.J. 1973. Regeneration of muscle. In: G.H. Bourne (ed.), *The Structure and Function of Muscle*, pp. 311-363. Acad. Press, New York-London.

Imamura, K. 1978. Ultrastructural aspect of left ventricular hypertrophy in spontaneously hypertensive rats: A qualitative and quantitative study. *Jap. Circ. J.* **42**:979-1002.

Laufer, A. 1971. Acute myocardial anoxia. Anatomical changes and their possible relation to immunological processes. *Cardiology* **56**:65-72.

Legato, M.J. 1972. Ultrastructural characteristics of the rat ventricular cell grown in tissue culture, with special reference to sarcomerogenesis. *J. Mol. Cell. Cardiol.* **4**:299-317.

Novi, A.M. 1968. Beitrag zur Feinstruktur des Herzmuskels bei experimenteller Herzhypertrophie. (The fine structure of myocardium in experimental heart hypertrophy.) *Beitr. path. Anat.* **137**:19-50.

Paniagua, R., Ceballos, L., and Vazquez. 1977. Reversible myocardial injury in rat by exhaustive exercise. *An. Anat.* **26**:317-332.

Ruff, S., and Strughold, H. 1957. *Grundriss der Luftfahrtmedizin.* (Compendium of Aviation Medicine.) J.A. Barth, Munich.

Turek, Z., Grandtner, M., and Kreuzer, F. 1972. Cardiac hypertrophy, capillary and muscle fiber density, muscle fiber diameter, capillary radius and diffusion distance in the myocardium of growing rats adapted to a simulated altitude of 3,500 m. *Pflugers Arch.* **335**:19-28.

Van Liere, E.J., and Stickney, J.C. 1963. *Hypoxia.* University of Chicago Press, Chicago.

Wachtlova, M., Mares, V., and Ostadal, B. 1977. DNA synthesis in the ventricular myocardium of young rats exposed to intermittent high altitude hypoxia. *Virchows Arch. B Cell Path.* **24**:335-342.

Effect of High Altitude Training on Muscle Enzyme Activities and Physical Performance Characteristics of Cross-Country Skiers

Paavo Rahkila and **Heikki Rusko**
University of Jyväskylä, Finland

Opinions differ concerning the question of whether or not performance at sea level is improved following an exposure to or training at high altitude. In well-trained athletes, some investigators have observed improved performance and increased maximum oxygen uptake on return to sea level, whereas others have found little or no effect after training at altitude (Banister and Woo, 1978; Buskirk et al., 1967; Daniels and Oldridge, 1970; Davies and Sargeant, 1974; Saltin, 1967). Using a control group, Adams et al (1975) found no potentiating effect on endurance performance or on maximum oxygen uptake in already well-trained middle distance runners when hard endurance training at 2,300 m was compared with equivalent training at sea level.

Increased activities of oxidative enzymes of muscle tissue have been found after altitude exposure in animals (Tenney, 1968; Weihe, 1966). The respiratory capacity of human muscle has been found to be apparently greater in altitude natives than in those at sea level (Reynafarje, 1962).

The purpose of this study was to evaluate the effects of a short cross-country skiing training camp at altitude on the physical performance characteristics and on the muscle enzyme activities of well-trained cross-country skiers.

Methods

Three groups of well-trained athletes were studied before and after a 3-week training period. One group of high altitude skiers (HAS, $n = 6$)

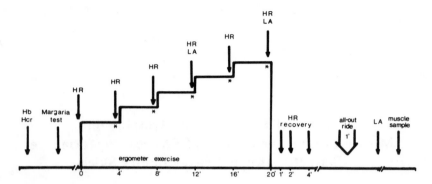

Figure 1—Schematic presentation of the testing procedure. (* = measurement of oxygen uptake).

trained 11 days at an altitude of 2,600 m in the middle of this period. Two other groups, called sea level skiers (SLS, $n = 8$) and sea level runners (SLR, $n = 6$), continued their training at sea level (100 m).

A schematic presentation of the various measurements is shown in Figure 1. Hemoglobin concentration (Hb) and hematocrit (Hcr) were estimated from capillary blood samples. Running speed was measured as vertical velocity (V_v) using the Margaria test.

A submaximal exercise test of 20 min. duration was used to estimate the aerobic performance capacity of the subjects. The subjects pedalled a Monark ergometer at 50 rpm and the intensity of exercise was increased every fourth minute. Lung ventilation (STPD) and oxygen uptake (STPD) were measured using a semiautomated system during the last minute of every 4 min. exercise period. Heart rate was calculated from an EKG recorded continuously during the exercise test and 4 min. after the test. Blood samples were taken from fingertips at the end of the 12th and 20th minute of exercise for the determination of blood lactate concentration (enzymatic method, Biochemica Boehringer). Maximum oxygen uptake was estimated from steady state heart rate and oxygen consumption values according to Andersen et al. (1971).

Thirty min. after the submaximal exercise test, the subjects performed a 1 min. all-out bicycle ergometer ride according to Szogy and Cherebetiu (1974). Muscular power was calculated as $kJ \times kg^{-1} \times min^{-1}$. A blood sample was taken from the fingertip 2.5 min. after the ride for the determination of lactate concentration.

Muscle samples from the vastus lateralis muscle were obtained using the needle biopsy technique after the exercise tests. Myosine ATPase staining was used to classify the muscle fibers as slow twitch (ST) and fast twitch (FT) types according to Gollnick et al. (1972). The following enzymatic activities were assayed: SDH, MDH, CS, and LDH. The

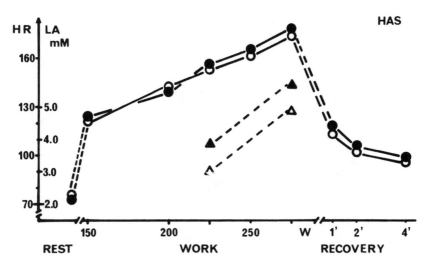

Figure 2—Heart rate (O, HR) and blood lactate (△, LA) response to incremental submaximal bicycle exercise in the group of high altitude skiers before (solid signs) and after (open signs) the training period.

specific enzyme activities were referred to protein content of the sample.

Results and Discussion

Table 1 shows that the SLS were taller than the others and that the HAS gained weight during the investigation period. The hemoglobin and hematocrit values of the HAS group increased significantly during the training period and the postvalues were significantly higher than those of the sea level groups. In other studies, elevated Hb-concentration was observed after only a few days' exposure at high altitude (e.g., Adams et al., 1975).

The heart rate during submaximal exercise was unaffected by high altitude training or by training at sea level. A slight, but not significant, reduction in blood lactate concentration was found in the HAS group (Figure 2). Lung ventilation (Figure 3) and oxygen uptake were reduced at three intensities of exercise in the HAS group. The estimated maximum oxygen uptake was not significantly changed in any group (Table 2). No significant changes were observed in vertical running velocity or in muscular power. The same was true for blood lactate values after a 1 min. all-out ride on a bicycle ergometer (Table 2).

Changes in the activities of muscle enzymes and in muscle fiber composition were insignificant (Figure 4). Similarly, none of the differences

Table 1—Anthropometric Data, Percentage of Slow Twitch Fibers (ST %), and Hemoglobin (Hb) and Hematocrit (Hcr) Values of the Groups Before (B) and After (A) the Training Period

Group	Height (cm)	ST (%)	Weight (kg)		Hb $g \times 1^{-1}$		Percentage of Hcr	
			B	A	B	A	B	A
HAS $\bar{x}$	174	55	66.3	67.7[a]	160	168[a]	47	49[a]
$n = 6$ s	5	11	2.8	2.8	15	11	3	4
SLS $\bar{x}$	179	58	74.4[b]	74.1[b]	150	149[b]	45	44[b]
$n = 8$ s	4	17	4.8	4.7	9	11	3	3
SLR $\bar{x}$	176	54	65.0	64.2	156	152[b]	48	45[b]
$n = 6$ s	4	16	4.7	4.4	2	5	3	2

[a]Significant change $p < 0.05$.
[b]Significant difference ($p < 0.05$) as compared with corresponding values of the HAS group.

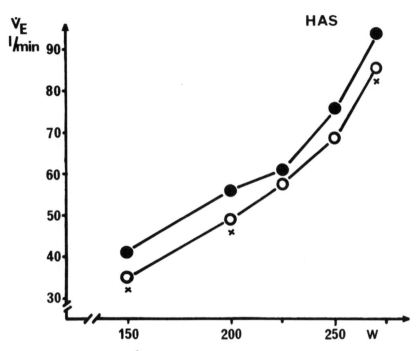

Figure 3—Lung ventilation ($\dot{V}_E$, STPD) during incremental submaximal bicycle exercise in the group of high altitude skiers before (solid signs) and after (open signs) the training period. The crosses indicate the significant differences ($p < 0.05$).

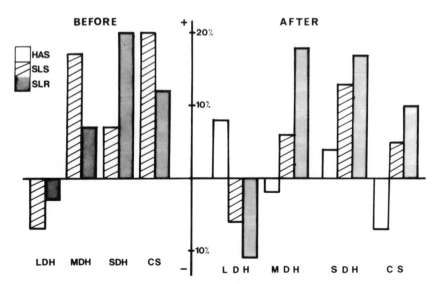

Figure 4—The relative changes and differences between groups in the activities of muscle enzymes. The base line indicates the mean value of each enzyme activity for the high altitude skiers before the training period.

Table 2—Estimated Maximum Oxygen Uptake (Max $\dot{V}_{O_2}$), Vertical Velocity (V_v), Muscular Power (MP), in and Blood Lactate (LA) After a 1-min. All-out Ride Before (B) and After (A) the Training Period

Group		Max $\dot{V}_{O_2}$ $l \times min^{-1}$ B	A	Max $\dot{V}_{O_2}$ $ml \times kg^{-1} \times min^{-1}$ B	A	V_v $m \times s^{-1}$ B	A	MP $kJ \times kg^{-1} \times min^{-1}$ B	A	LA $mM \times l^{-1}$ B	A
HAS	$\bar{x}$	4.4	4.3	66	64	1.36	1.38	422	422	10.9	12.5
	s	0.2	0.5	4	6	0.12	0.08	27	26	1.8	1.7
SLS	$\bar{x}$	4.6	4.6	62	62	1.42	1.37	412	412	12.8	13.9
	s	0.4	0.4	7	6	0.10	0.08	26	25	1.5	2.1
SLR	$\bar{x}$	4.1	4.0	63	62	1.38	1.42	432	441	10.6	11.9
	s	0.4	0.3	4	6	0.07	0.05	29	39	2.6	1.3

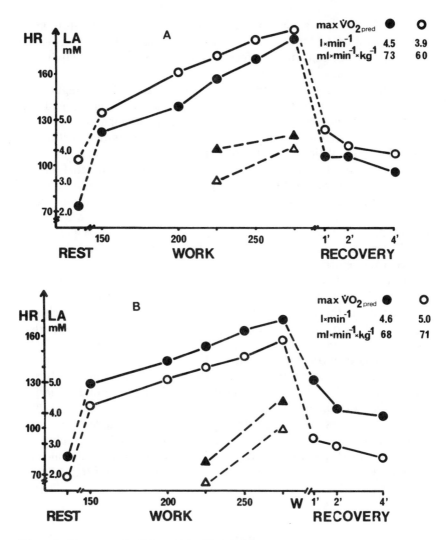

Figure 5—Heart rate (O, HR) and blood lactate ($\triangle$, LA) response to submaximal exercise for two HAS subjects (A and B) before (solid signs) and after (open signs) the training period.

between the groups before or after the training period was significant. The groups which trained at sea level tended to have higher activities of oxidative enzymes and lower LDH activity than the HAS group, both before and after the training period. An increase in hemoglobin concentration and in hematocrit can be considered as an indication of hypoxic stress at altitude; however, training at high altitude together with this hypoxic stress had no potentiating effect on muscle enzyme activities as compared with equivalent training at sea level. Although the altitude exposure was short and the subjects were well-trained athletes, it seems that hypoxia does not explain the effect of endurance training on activities of oxidative enzymes.

Individual results in Figure 5 show that Subject A had a higher and Subject B a lower heart rate at rest, during submaximal exercise, and during recovery after the training period. Their estimated maximum oxygen uptakes were correspondingly changed. Both subjects demonstrated a small decrease in blood lactate concentration during submaximal exercise. During the investigation period, these subjects competed equally well, but afterwards, Subject B competed far more successfully in ski races. It seems evident that Subject A had lost his fitness after the training camp at high altitude. In our study, two of the six skiers who trained for 11 days at altitude improved their performance, two performed equally well, and two demonstrated a definite impairment in their performance after returning to sea level.

Short ski training camps at altitude belong nowadays to the training regimen of almost all elite cross-country skiers of the world during summertime and in the autumn. According to the present results, these training camps may be more beneficial for improving skiing techniques than for purposes of physiological adaptation. The duration and intensity of training may be more important than the hypoxic stress. Nevertheless, it may be easier to disturb the homeostasis of bodily functions at altitude than at sea level. This may explain the improvements found in performance and in some physiological parameters after training at high altitude in studies without control groups. It is concluded that more follow-up studies on highly trained athletes are needed to establish the reasons for the apparently diverse individual adaptations to high altitude training, which has also been mentioned in other studies (e.g., Saltin, 1967).

References

Adams, W.C., Bernauer, E.M., Dill, D.B., and Bomar, J.B.Jr. 1975. Effects of equivalent sea-level and altitude training on $\dot{V}_{O_2}$max and running performance. *J. Appl. Physiol.* **39**:262-266.

Andersen, K.L., Shephard, R., Denolin, H., Varnauskas, E., and Masironi, R. 1971. *Fundamentals of Exercise Testing.* World Health Organization, Geneva.

Banister, E.W., and Woo, W. 1978. Effects of simulated altitude training on aerobic and anaerobic power. *Eur. J. Appl. Physiol.* **38**:55-69.

Buskirk, E.R., Kollias, J., Piconreatique, E., Akers, R., Prokop, E., and Baker, P. 1967. Physiology and performance of track athletes at various altitudes in the United States and Peru. In: *The International Symposium on the Effects of*

Altitude on Physical Performance, pp. 65-72. The Athletic Institute. Albuquerque, NM.

Daniels, J., and Oldridge, N. 1970. The effects of alternate exposure to altitude and sea level on world-class middle-distance runners. *Med. Sci. Sports.* 2:107-112.

Davies, C.T.M., and Sargeant, A.J. 1974. Effects of hypoxic training on normoxic maximal aerobic power output. *Eur. J. Appl. Physiol.* 33:854-859.

Gollnick, P., Armstrong, R., Saubert, C., Piehl, K., and Saltin, B. 1972. Enzyme activity and fiber composition in skeletal muscle of untrained and trained men. *J. Appl. Physiol.* 33:312-319.

Reynafarje, B. 1962. Myoglobin content and enzymatic activity of muscle and altitude adaption. *J. Appl. Physiol.* 17:301-305.

Saltin, B. 1967. Aerobic and anaerobic work capacity at an altitude of 2,250 meters. In: *The International Symposium on the Effects of Altitude on Physical Performance*, pp. 97-102. The Athletic Institute, Albuquerque, NM.

Szogy, A., and Cherebetiu, G. 1974. Minutentest auf dem Fahrradergometer zur Bestimmung der anaeroben Kapazitat. (A 1-min. bicycle ergometer test for determination of anerobic capacity.) *Eur. J. Appl. Physiol.* 33:171-176.

Tenney, S.M. 1968. Physiological adaptations to life at high altitude. In: E. Jokl and P. Jokl (eds.), *Medicine and Sport.* Vol. 1., Exercise and Altitude, pp. 60-70. S. Karger, Basel, Switzerland.

Weihe, W.H. 1966. Time course of adaptation to different altitudes at tissue level. *Schweiz. Z. Sportmed.* 14:177-190.

Physical Performance as a Function of Liquid Intake

H.U. Wanner
Swiss Federal Institute of Technology, Zurich, Switzerland

Sportsmen and their coaches are often confronted with the problem of nutrition during the period of training and during competition. In recent years, the question of liquid intake during a continuous performance has been of special interest. Recent investigations have shown that dehydration causes a reduction in performance and disturbs thermoregulation. Sufficient liquid intake before and during a continuous performance is necessary to reduce the loss of performance and to prevent negative health effects (Costill, 1978; Franz and Franz, 1978; Gebert, 1978).

In four different studies, performed by students for their theses (Fasser-Marti, 1978; Frei, 1979; Gmunder, 1979; Wahli, 1979), the following problems were investigated:

1. Weight loss during physical performance in relation to temperature (15, 20, and 25 °C) and liquid intake;

2. Performance loss in relation to liquid intake;

3. Heart rate fluctuation (with and without liquid intake) during "aerobic" performance, "anaerobic" performance, and pauses;

4. Effect of the additives "Isostar" and "Gatorade"—as compared with that of water.

Methods

All tests were carried out either in a climatic chamber or in a gymnastic hall at constant temperature and relative humidity. The tests were performed on bicycle ergometers; the loads varied between 120 and 320 Watt, the time of performance varied between 1½ and 2 hr. The heart rate was continuously monitored with a cardiometer or a telemetric unit. Liquid was taken every 5 or 10 min.; amounts varied between 0.75 and 1.5 dL. Each subject was tested with and without liquid intake.

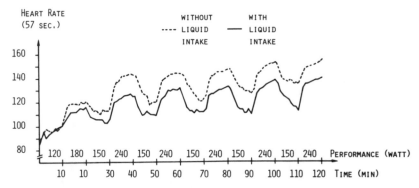

Figure 1—"Aerobic" performance at high and low levels during 2 hr. Heart rates with and without liquid intake; values of an individual subject. Liquid intake: 1.5 dL water every 10 min.

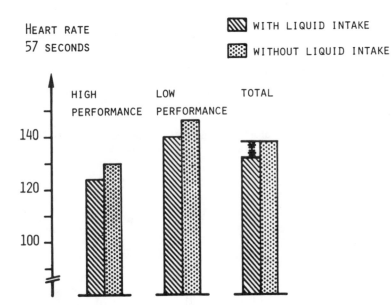

Figure 2—"Aerobic" performance alternately at high and low levels during 2 hr. Heart rates with and without liquid intake. Average of 10 subjects. Liquid intake: 1.5 dL water every 10 minutes. **$p < 0.01$.

Results

Figures 1-6 illustrate some of the most important results. Further details are given in the four studies mentioned (Fasser-Marti, 1978; Frei, 1979; Gmunder, 1979; Wahli, 1979).

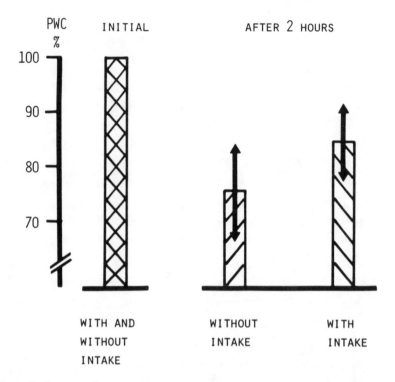

Figure 3—Decrease of an "aerobic" performance of 2 hr. with and without liquid intake. Values based on the physical work capacity (PWC 170). Average of 10 subjects.

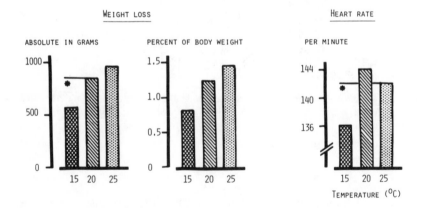

Figure 4—Liquid loss and heart rate as a function of temperature. "Aerobic" performance during 1 hr. Average of six subjects. $*p < 0.05$.

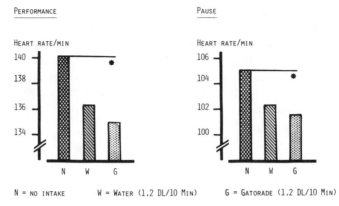

PERFORMANCE

PAUSE

Figure 5—"Aerobic" performance during 2 hr. (in 12 consecutive phases: 8 min. for performance and 2 min. for pauses). Heart rates with and without liquid intake—average of 10 subjects. *$p < 0.05$.

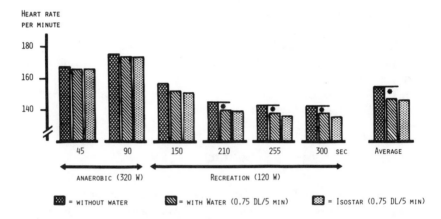

Figure 6—"Anaerobic" performance—average of six consecutive time phases of 300 sec. Heart rates with and without liquid intake—average of eight subjects (racing cyclists). *$p < 0.05$.

The four studies showed very similar effects: With regular liquid intake—1 to 1.5 dL. every 10 min.—the heart rate was, on the average, six to eight beats per minute lower than without liquid supply. There were individual differences: heart rates were in general lower in the cases of those test persons who were accustomed to the regular intake of liquid during the physical performance. The weight losses were lower at a temperature of 15 °C than at 20 and 25 °C. There was a correlation between reduction of weight through loss of liquid and decrease in physical performance.

From these results and those of comparable investigations we can draw the following conclusions:

Regular liquid intake in cases of 45-60 min. performance results in: (a) lower loss of weight and performance, (b) lower increment of heart rate, and (c) quicker recovery after "aerobic" and "anaerobic" performances. These differences could be due to a lower load on circulation, a lower reduction in volume of plasma, and a better temperature regulation.

Recommendations

According to the results of the performed tests and further investigation, the following concrete proposals can be made:

1. Liquid intake should be provided in the case of continuous performances of more than 45 min.

2. Regular intervals of 10 to 20 min. should be maintained.

3. Intake should be in small portions up to 2 dL.

4. In cases of continuous performance of more than 1½ to 2 hr., glucose and electrolytes should be added to the liquid.

5. Liquid should be taken ½ to 1 hr. before the start of a continuous performance.

6. The intake of liquid should be regular, the amount and the frequency depending upon the type of discipline.

Summary

In four experimental studies, the influence of dehydration and liquid intake on the physical performance was investigated. Tests were performed under controlled conditions on a bicycle ergometer. The variables were intake of drinking water or water with electrolytes, and the environmental temperature. The heart rate was continuously registered. The results showed that with regular liquid intake the heart rate was on the average 6-8 beats per minute lower than without liquid supply. The heart rates were in general lower in those test persons who were accustomed to the regular intake of liquid during continuous performance. There was a correlation between reduction of weight due to loss of liquid and decrease in physical performance.

Acknowledgments

The work of Magdalena Fasser-Marti, Evelyne Frei, Gabriela Wahli, and A.

Gmunder and the help of R. Gierer for technical assistance are thankfully acknowledged. Special thanks to Dr. P.J. Jenoure, who was consulted during these studies.

References

Costill, D.L. 1978. *Pourquoi et que boire au cours de l'exercise prolongé?* Reproduction of "The New Runner's Diet" by permission of World Publications, Mountain View, CA.

Fasser-Marti, M. 1978. *Einfluss von Flussigkeitsverlust und Flussigkeitszufuhr auf das Dauerleistungsvermogen.* (Influence of liquid loss and liquid supply upon the ability of endurance performance.) Diploma work, Courses gymnastics and sport, ETH Zurich.

Franz, G., and Franz, I.-W. 1978. Untersuchungen uber die Flussigkeitsverluste und deren Substitution bei einem Volksmarathonlauf. (Investigations of the liquid losses and their substitution during marathon.) *Deutsche Zeitschrift fuer Sportmedizin*, **29**(6):165-172.

Frei, E. 1979. *Flussigkeitsverlust bei Ausdauerleistungen in Abhangigkeit der Temperatur.* (Liquid loss during continuing performances depending on the temperature.) Diploma work, Courses gymnastics and sport, ETH Zurich.

Gebert, G. 1978. Probleme des Wasser-Temperature- und Elektrolythaushaltes beim Sportler. (Problems concerning the water/temperature and the electrolytical economy for athletes.) *Deutsche Zeitschrift fuer Sportmedizin* **29**(6):159-165.

Gmunder, A. 1979. *Die Bedeutung der Zufuhr von Flussigkeit, Nahrstoffen und Electrolyten bei Ausdauersportlern.* (The importance of liquid, nutritive substances and electrolyte supply for endurance athletes.) Diploma work, Courses gymnastics and sport, ETH Zurich.

Wahli, G. 1979. *Flussigkeits- und Elektrolytenzufuhr bei Dauerleistungen. Untersuchungen mit Radrennfahrern.* (Liquid and electrolyte supply for endurance performances. Investigations with racing cyclists.) Diploma work, Courses gymnastics and sport, ETH Zurich.

Physical Performance Characteristics
of the Finnish National Ice Hockey Team

M. Vainikka, P. Rahkila, and **H. Rusko**
Research Unit for Sport and Physical Fitness, Finland

Intermittent work is typical of ice hockey. The findings of heart rate (Forsberg et al., 1974; Green et al., 1978), oxygen uptake (Patterson, 1979), blood lactate concentration (Green et al., 1976), and muscle glycogen depletion (Montpetit et al., 1979) during actual or simulated play situations indicate the intensive nature of the performances involved in ice hockey. The anaerobic portion of the metabolism during one shift has been demonstrated to be about 65-70% of the total energy expenditure (Seliger et al., 1972). Laboratory investigations indicate that ice hockey players have lower maximum oxygen uptake and higher blood lactate concentration after maximal exercise test than endurance athletes (Forsberg et al. 1974; Komi et al. 1977; Leger et al. 1979).

The purpose of this study was to describe the physical performance characteristics of the Finnish National Ice Hockey Team.

Methods

The Finnish National Ice Hockey Team ($n = 27$) studied consisted of 3 goaltenders, 8 defensemen, and 16 forwards. The age of the subjects varied from 18.4 to 29.9 years ($\overline{X} = 23.9$; SD $= 2.6$ years), and they had played continuously on the national team an average of 1.6 years. The measurements were carried out in August, 1978. Before the study, details of the measurements and the associated risks were described to the subjects, and their written consent to participate was obtained.

The following anthropometric variables were determined: height, weight, and the percentage of body fat (% F) by skinfold measurements (Durnin and Rahaman, 1967). In order to determine maximum oxygen uptake (max $\dot{V}_{O_2}$) and the anaerobic threshold (AT) of the subjects, an incremental bicycle ergometer (Monark) exercise was carried out. The friction force was increased every 2nd minute up to exhaustion, which occurred after about 20 min. The pedalling frequency (60 rpm) was recorded by an electronic counter. Lung ventilation (VE, STPD), oxygen uptake ($\dot{V}_{CO_2}$) were measured continuously for every 40 sec. period during the exercise by a semiautomated system (Rusko et al., 1980). Blood samples for the enzymatic analysis of the lactate concentration (LA) were taken from fingertips at the 6th, 10th, 14th, 18th min. of the exercise as well as 0.5 and 2.5 min. after exhaustion. Heart rate (HR) was calculated from ECG registered (Mingograph 14) every minute.

The greatest values of power (P), $\dot{V}E$, $\dot{V}_{O_2}$, HR, and LA were considered as maximum for each subject. To determine the anaerobic threshold, $\dot{V}E$ and $\dot{V}_{CO_2}$ were plotted against the corresponding $\dot{V}_{O_2}$-and HR-values. Departure from linearity in the respiratory responses was used as a criterion of anaerobic threshold. The increase of blood lactate concentration over about 4 mM was used together with the respiratory responses to verify that AT had been reached (Rusko et al., 1980).

The running speed (vertical velocity) of the subjects was measured according to Margaria et al. (1966). The muscular performance of the players was measured during two 1 min. all-out rides on a bicycle ergometer (Monark) (Szogy and Cherebetiu, 1974). The bicycle ergometer-rides were separated by a 3-min. recovery period. Blood samples for enzymatic analysis of LA were taken from fingertips 2.5 min. after both bicycle ergometer-rides.

The measurements were carried out in the following order: running speed, anthropometry, incremental bicycle ergometry, and two all-out bicycle ergometer-rides.

Standard procedures were used to calculate means and standard deviations. The Student's t-test (2P) was used to analyze the differences between the player groups.

Results

The anthropometric characteristics of the subjects are presented in Table 1. Defensemen and forwards were, on the average, taller than the goaltenders. But the differences among player groups were not significant.

During the incremental bicycle ergometer-test, the subjects obtained, on the average, the maximum power of 296 W, max HR of 187 beats · min^{-1}, max $\dot{V}_{O_2}$ of 52 ml · kg^{-1} min^{-1}, max $\dot{V}E$ of 119 liters · min^{-1} and max LA of 12.1 mM (Table 2). The anaerobic threshold was ob-

Table 1— Anthropometric Characteristics of Subjects ($\overline{X}$ ± S.D.)

Variable	Goaltenders (n = 3)	Defensemen (n = 8)	Forwards (n = 16)	Overall (n = 27)
Height (cm)	177.9 ± 6.0	180.2 ± 6.5	180.0 ± 4.3	179.9 ± 5.0
Weight (kg)	77.4 ± 5.4	82.9 ± 6.6	81.5 ± 6.3	81.1 ± 6.0
Percentage of F	13.0 ± 3.6	12.0 ± 1.5	13.6 ± 2.9	13.0 ± 2.6

Table 2—Results of the Incremental Bicycle Ergometer Test ($\overline{X}$ ± S.D.)

Variable	Goaltenders (n = 3)	Defensemen (n = 8)	Forwards (n = 16)	Overall (n = 27)
max P (W)	266.0 ± 41.0	297.0 ± 26.0	302.0 ± 22.0	296.0 ± 26.0
max $\dot{V}_{O_2}$ (l·min^{-1})	3.7 ± 0.7	4.4 ± 0.6	4.3 ± 0.4	4.3 ± 0.5
max $\dot{V}_{O_2}$ (ml·kg^{-1}·min^{-1})	47.0 ± 7.0	53.0 ± 6.0	53.0 ± 7.0	52.0 ± 6.0
max $\dot{V}E$ (l·min^{-1})	104.0 ± 16.0	128.0 ± 18.0	117.0 ± 17.0	119.0 ± 18.0
max HR (beats·min^{-1})	187.0 ± 10.0	185.0 ± 5.0	187.0 ± 8.0	187.0 ± 7.0
max LA (mM)	11.3 ± 4.3	12.9 ± 2.0	11.8 ± 2.5	12.1 ± 2.5
AT (W)	213.0 ± 35.0	240.0 ± 18.0	237.0 ± 23.0	235.0 ± 23.0
AT $\dot{V}_{O_2}$ (ml·kg^{-1}·min^{-1})	34.0 ± 7.0	37.0 ± 3.0	38.0 ± 5.0	38.0 ± 5.0
AT HR (beats·min^{-1})	161.0 ± 14.0	162.0 ± 6.0	162.0 ± 11.0	162.0 ± 10.0

served at the mean power of 235 W (79% of maximum), corresponding to HR of 162 beats · min^{-1} (76% of max HR), and $\dot{V}_{O_2}$ of 38 ml · kg^{-1} · min^{-1} (68% of max $\dot{V}_{O_2}$). The goaltenders tended to have lower values (p < .05) when compared to defensemen and forwards.

The mean vertical velocity of the subjects was 1.58 ± 0.10 m · sec^{-1}. No significant differences were found between the groups (Table 3).

The results of the two 1 min. all-out bicycle ergometer-rides are presented in Table 3. During the first bicycle ergometer-ride, the defensemen (396 J · kg^{-1}) attained higher (p < .05) mean power when compared to the goaltenders (368 J · kg^{-1}). No other significant differences were found between the player groups. During the second ride, the mean power decreased significantly to 83-87% of that of the first ride. Blood lactate concentration after the bicycle ergometer-rides increased significantly from 13.8 to 17.6 mM (Table 3.).

Table 3—Results of the Margaria Test
and the Two (I, II) All-out Bicycle Ergometer Rides ($\overline{X}$ ± S.D.)

Variable		Goaltenders ($n = 3$)	Defensemen ($n = 8$)	Forwards ($n = 16$)	Overall ($n = 27$)
Vertical velocity (m·sec^{-1})		1.53 ± .12	1.61 ± .10	1.58 ± .10	1.58 ± .10
All-out bicycle ergometer rides					
Amount of work (J·kg^{-1})	I	366 ± 12	396 ± 18	379 ± 24	383 ± 24
	II	318 ± 30	330 ± 24	330 ± 18	326 19
HR (b·min^{-1})	I	178 ± 12	172 ± 7	173 ± 6	173 ± 7
	II	186 ± 7	174 ± 4	177 ± 7	177 ± 7
LA (mM)	I	14.3 ± 2.2	14.4 ± 1.9	13.4 ± 1.0	13.8 ± 1.5
	II	17.7 ± 1.5	18.6 ± 1.5	17.1 ± 2.2	17.6 ± 2.0

Discussion

The height, weight, and percentage of fat of the subjects were almost equal when compared to other ice hockey teams studied (Forsberg et al., 1974; Green et al., 1979; Liesen et al., 1977; Seliger et al., 1972). The players were taller when compared with other Finnish elite athletes (Rusko et al., 1978). The tallness can partly be explained by the selection of the players, because the ability to exert force against external objects (e.g., an opponent in contact situations) depends on body size.

Previous studies have shown that elite ice hockey requires high aerobic and anaerobic power (for references, see Green, 1979; Montpetit et al., 1979). By taking into account both the methodological (bicycle vs. treadmill exercise) and the seasonal differences of the measurements between the studies, it can be estimated that max $\dot{V}_{O_2}$ (52 ml · kg^{-1} kg^{-1} · min^{-1}) and anaerobic threshold (38 ml · kg^{-1} · min^{-1}) of the Finnish players is almost equal when compared to Swedish, Czech, German, and Canadian players (Table 4).

Vertical velocity, which has been used as an indicator of anaerobic alactic power, was lower in the Finnish players (1.58 m · sec^{-1}) when compared with Canadian players (1.69 m · sec^{-1}; Green and Houston, 1975). The low running speed of the Finnish ice hockey players has also been reported by Komi et al. (1977). These results may be due to the higher proportion of slow twitch muscle fibers in the thigh muscles of the Finnish players (Rusko et al., 1978) as compared with Canadian (Green et al., 1979) or Swedish (Forsberg et al., 1974) players.

Table 4—Max $\dot{V}_{O_2}$ and Anaerobic Threshold of Ice Hockey Players According to Some Studies ($\bar{X}$)

Nationality	(n)	Max $\dot{V}_{O_2}$ $l{\cdot}min^{-1}$	Max $\dot{V}_{O_2}$ $ml{\cdot}kg^{-1}{\cdot}min^{-1}$	Anaerobic Threshold $ml{\cdot}kg^{-1}{\cdot}min^{-1}$	Anaerobic Threshold HR	References
Canadian[b]	( )	—	54	39	—	Wenger et al., 1979
Czech[a]	(13)	4.32	55	—	—	Seliger et al., 1972
Finnish[a]	(27)	4.27	52	38	162	This study
German[a]	(9)	4.24	54	44	172	Liesen et al., 1974
Swedish[b]	(24)	4.31	57	—	—	Forsberg et al., 1974

Note. [a]Bicycle ergometer, [b]Treadmill

The blood lactate concentrations after the 1 min. all-out bicycle ergometer-rides (Table 3) indicate that the Finnish players had an equal or even higher anaerobic lactate capacity than Canadian players (Green, 1978; Green and Houston, 1975).

Previous studies indicate that during every shift of the play the heart rate of the players is 80% of max HR and that oxygen consumption is higher than 70% of max $\dot{V}_{O_2}$ (Forsberg et al., 1974; Green et al., 1978). In the present study, the anaerobic threshold of the subjects was observed at HR of 162 b · min^{-1} (76% of max HR) and at oxygen uptake of (38 ml · kg^{-1} · min^{-1} (68% of max $\dot{V}_{O_2}$), on the average. Thus, it seems that the players have to play at a higher power than AT. This was observed as increased blood lactate concentration during the actual play situations (Forsberg et al., 1974; Green et al., 1978). Because the determination of AT is based on the onset of steep accumulation of blood lactate, only small changes in the intensity of exercise appear as large changes in blood lactate concentration. Hence, only minor improvements in max $\dot{V}_{O_2}$ and AT may result in considerable decrease in blood lactate during the shift. Similarly, if two teams with different aerobic potentials are playing against each other, the team with weaker potentials is forced to play, on the average, at a higher relative power, e.g., at a higher heart rate and higher lactate concentration. Actually, Forsberg et al. (1974) have shown that heart rate and blood lactate concentration during play vary according to the opposing team.

In addition to the accumulation of lactate, influence of the low max $\dot{V}_{O_2}$ and AT can be demonstrated as increased utilization of muscle glycogen stores when working at equal intensity. The depletion of muscle glycogen has been shown to induce fatigue and decrease high level performance during the course of the contest. Playing ice hockey demands the precise coordination of several muscle groups which are superimposed on skating activity. Lactate accumulation and glycogen depletion may lead to a loss of control in skating and a deterioration of the skilled movement patterns of the upper body.

In conclusion, it seems clear that the overall tempo of ice hockey play is determined by the maximal oxygen uptake and the anaerobic threshold of the players. A heavy involvement of ATP and CP utilization and ATP reformation via glycolysis may be necessary in particular play situations. The Finnish National Team studied possessed a well-developed anaerobic lactate capacity; however, the potential of the aerobic system as reflected in central (max $\dot{V}_{O_2}$) and peripheral (AT) adaptations was equal or even worse as compared with foreign teams. Special programs to improve the aerobic characteristic of the players should therefore be developed.

References

Durnin, J., and Rahaman, M. 1976. The assessment of the amount of fat in the human body from measurement of skinfold thickness. *Brit. J. Nutr.* 21:681-689.

Forsberg, A., Hulten, B., Wilson, G., and Karlsson, J. 1974. *Ishockey. Idrottsfysiologi rapport* nr 14. (Ice Hockey: Sport Physiology Report No. 14.) Trygg-Hansa Forlagsverksamheten, Stockholm.

Green, H. 1979. Metabolic aspects of intermittent work with specific regard to ice hockey. *Canad. J. Appl. Sport Sci.* 4:29-34.

Green, H. 1978. Glycogen depletion patterns during continuous and intermittent ice skating. *Med. Sci. Sports* 10:183-187.

Green, H., and Houston, M. 1975. Effects of a season of ice hockey on energy capacities and associated functions. *Med. Sci. Sports* 7:299-303.

Green, H., Bishop, P., Houston, M., McKillip, R., Norman, R., and Stothart, P. 1976. Time motion and physiological assessments of ice hockey performance. *J. Appl. Physiol.* 40:159-163.

Green, H., Daub, W., Painter, D., and Thomson, J. 1978. Glycogen depletion patterns during ice hockey performance. *Med. Sci. Sports* 10:289-293.

Green, H., Thomson, J., Daub, W., Houston, M., and Ranney, D. 1979. Fibre composition, fibre size and enzyme activities in vastus lateralis of elite athletes involved in high intensity exercise. *Europ. J. Appl. Physiol.* 41:109-117.

Komi, P.V., Rusko, H., Vos, J., and Vihko, V. 1977. Anaerobic performance capacity in athletes. *Acta Physical. Scand.* 100:107-114.

Leger, L., Seliger, V., and Bassarel, L. 1979. Comparison among V_{O_2}-values for hockey players and runners. *Canad. J. Appl. Sport Sci.* 4:18-21.

Liesen, H., Mader, A., Heck, H., and Hollman, W. 1977. Die Ausdauerleistungsfahigkeit bei verschiedenen Sportarten under besouderer Berucksichtigung des Metabolismus: zur Ermittlung der optimalen Belastungsintensitat im Training. (The ability for endurance performance in various sport disciplines with special regard to the metabolism: For determination of the optimal loading intensity during training.). *Beiheft zu Leistungsport* 9:63-79.

Margaria, R., Aghemo, P., and Rovelli, E. 1966. Measurement of muscular power (anaerobic) in man. *J. Appl. Physiol.* 21(5):166-1664.

Montpetit, R., Binette, P., and Taylor, A. 1979. Glycogen depletion in a game-simulated hockey task. *Canad. J. Appl. Sport Sci.* 4:43-45.

Paterson, D. 1979. Respiratory and cardiovascular aspects of intermittent exercise with regard to ice hockey. *Canad. J. Appl. Sport Sci.* 4:22-28.

Rusko, H., Havu, M., and Karvinen, E. 1978. Aerobic performance capacity in athletes. *Europ. J. Appl. Physiol.* 38:151-159.

Rusko, H., Rahkila, P., and Karvinen, E. 1980. Anaerobic threshold, skeletal muscle enzymes and fiber composition in young female cross-country skiers. Acta Physiol. Scand. 108:263-268.

Seliger, V., Kostka, V., Grusova, D., Kovac, J., Machovcova, J., Pauer, M., Pribylova, A., and Urbankova, K. 1972. Energy expenditure and physical fitness of ice hockey players. *Int. Z. agnew. Physiol.* 30:283-291.

Szogy, A., and Cherebetiu, G. 1974. Minutentest auf dem Fahrradergometer zur Bestimmung der anaeroben Kapazitat. (1-minute test on the bicycle ergometer to determine anaerobic capacity.) *Europ. J. Appl. Physiol.* **43**:171-176.
Wenger, H., Quinney, H., Smith, D., Sexsmith, J., Thoms, J., and Drake, C. 1979. Physiological profiles of the Canadian Olympic hockey team. *Canad. J. Appl. Sport Sci.* **4**:246.

Horizontal Velocity Changes of
World-Class Skiers Using the Diagonal Technique

P.V. Komi
University of Jyväskylä, Finland

R.W. Norman and **G. Caldwell**
University of Waterloo, Canada

The mechanisms of propulsion in cross-country skiing are not well documented although informed speculations appear in many ski manuals and are promoted by instructors and coaches. An extensive temporal and kinematic analysis of world-class skiers has recently been published (Mietk et al., 1978). This will undoubtedly assist in producing the required objective information; however, selected body positions of the skiers, rather than the complete time histories of their movement cycles, were studied. The ideal way to approach the problem is to measure the time histories of forces and their phasic relationships from instrumented poles and skiis using telemetry; this is expensive, however.

A method which is less satisfactory than a direct force analysis, but which provides somewhat more information about propulsion mechanisms than that used by Mietk et al. (1978), is to calculate the instantaneous position of the center of gravity of the skier and to create a horizontal velocity/time profile over a step cycle. Changes in the velocity can then be related to relative angular displacement and velocity profiles of the hips, knees, ankles, and other joints which can contribute to propulsion.

Methods

Most of the competitors in the men's 15 km race at the 1978 World Championships in Lahti, Finland, were filmed by a joint research team of Finns, Swiss, and Canadians, using 16mm cameras at a rate of 60

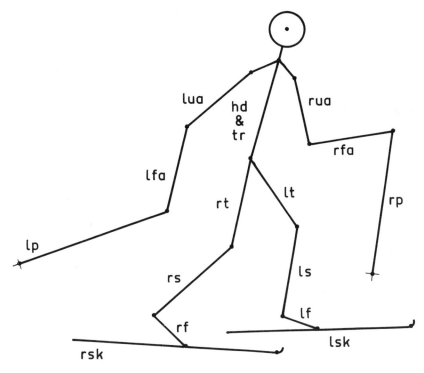

Figure 1—Linked segment model of skier.

frames per second. The films were taken on a relatively flat position of the course about 9.4 km into the race. The elevation at this point was 23 cm in 6.5 m (approximately 3.5%) and the competitors were using the diagonal technique.

Fifteen segment models, including skis and poles (Figure 1), of five skiers were created by digitizing appropriate end points on a computer interfaced Numonics film analyzer. The coordinates were smoothed using a second order low pass Butterworth digital filter at a cutoff frequency of 4.5 Hz (Pezzack et al. 1977; Winter et al. 1974). The time histories of the linear displacement, velocity and acceleration of each digitized point, i.e. body joint, center of gravity of each segment, and the total body center of gravity were calculated for one step, using a finite difference technique (Miller and Nelson, 1973) on the filtered data. The absolute and relative angular displacement, velocity, and acceleration profiles of each segment and joint in the model were also generated.

Table 1—Skier Information

Skier	JL	JM	MP	PV	KS
Race finish	1	3	4	32	58
Race time	49:09.8	49:14:4	49:23.9	51:46.8	54:33.0
Weight (kg)	67	94	71	70	65
Height (cm)	173	196	176	174	176

Table 2—Kinematic Data

Skier	JL	JM	MP	PV	KS
Step velocity (m/s)	4.70	4.86	4.83	4.76	4.91
Step length (m)	2.90	3.20	3.10	2.80	2.80
Step time (s)	.62	.65	.64	.59	.57

Results

Complete data were obtained on five skiers. The skiers place of finish and time are summarized in Table 1. Only 14 sec. separated the first and fourth finishers and only 5 min. and 24 sec. separated first and 58th place. This is 0.5 and 11%, respectively in a race which ended in about 50 min.

Some basic temporal and kinematic data appear in Table 2. The average horizontal velocity of the center of gravity over the step was 4.81 m/s (range 4.70-4.91 m/s). This was produced by an average step length of 2.96m (range 2.8-3.2m) and average step time of 0.61s (range 0.57-0.65s) or average step rate of 1.63 steps/s.

Examples of individual horizontal velocity curves during one step are seen in Figures 2 and 3. These curves begin at an arbitrary point in the step cycle, where the trailing leg is just beginning its return. This is called "End of Kick of the Right or Left Leg" (EKR, EKL, respectively). One complete step and gait cycle is therefore EKL to EKR or vice versa. Other symbols are defined in the figure captions. In general, the curves show three periods of increasing velocity: (a) shortly following pole plant and probably attributable to the use of the pole and/or the momentum of the forward swinging recovery leg, as suggested by Gagnon (1980), while it begins to decelerate; (b) shortly after the legs come together, attributable to the combined leg and pole push but of unknown proportion of each;

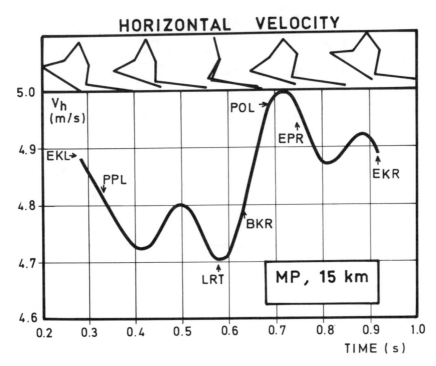

Figure 2—Horizontal velocity of body center of gravity during 1 step. Skier MP. EKL, EKR = end of follow-through of trail leg, left or right; PPL, PPR = pole plant left, right; BKL, BKR = beginning of kick of left (right) leg; POL, POR = pole just taken off the ground left, right; EPL, EPR = end of push of left (right) leg.

(c) just before the end of the "kick", during glide, possibly attributable to the upward deceleration of the trailing leg and rising trunk. This would have a momentary effect of reducing the weight on the gliding ski, thus reducing the retarding frictional force.

Interestingly, the largest velocity increase occurred during leg and pole push (about 0.3 m/s) for skier MP in Figure 2. With skier KS, however (Figure 3), the largest velocity increase, also about 0.3 m/s, occurred shortly following pole plant during the forward swing of the recovery leg. A further sizable increase of 0.1 m/s occurred during leg and pole push.

Indeed, if these curves for the five subjects are normalized to percentage of step time and superimposed, the details of the patterns of velocity change are similar for three skiers but somewhat different for the other two (Figure 4). They are all skiing fast, but they appear to be achieving their speed in different ways. The maximum velocity change on the average was 0.31 m/s (range 0.21-0.40 m/s) and occurred during the leg push phase for three skiers but during the free leg swing/pole push phase for

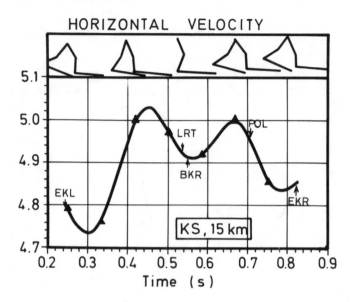

Figure 3—Horizontal velocity of body center of gravity during 1 step. Skier KS. See Figure 2 for symbols.

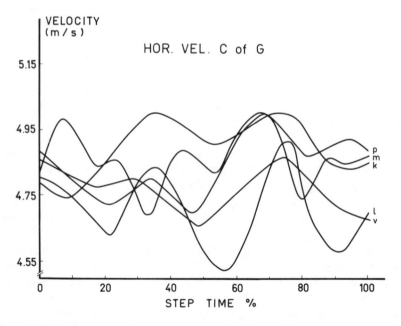

Figure 4—Horizontal velocity of body center of gravity of five skiers normalized to percentage of single step time.

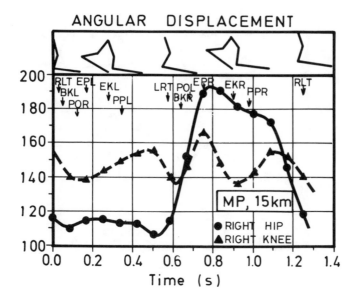

Figure 5—Relative angular displacement of hip and knee joint during one complete stride (two steps). Skier MP. See Figure 2 for symbols.

two skiers. It is apparent from Figure 4 that attempting to average the horizontal velocity of the center of gravity amplitudes to produce an "average" pattern would result in an unrealistic curve.

Hip and Knee Joint Kinematics

Some evidence as to the use of the hip and knee joints, particularly during push, can be found in the relative angular displacement and velocity curves. Figures 5 and 6 are angular displacement curves for MP and KS, respectively. Note that these curves show a complete stride rather than a single step.

Skier MP goes through a range of motion of about 85° from a hip joint angle of 107° to a hyperextension of 192° during leg push. Skier KS extends his hip joint from 111 to 183° for a 72° range of motion.

The knee joint extension during leg push goes from 136 to 165° or a range of motion of 29° for MP. KS, on the other hand, extends from 131 to 155°, a 24° range of motion. Both skiers exhibit a slight flexion at both the hip and knee just prior to extension.

Even more important than the range of motion of the hip and knee joints is the velocity at which the movements occur. Figures 7 and 8 show the angular velocity curves for skiers MP and KS, respectively. Extension

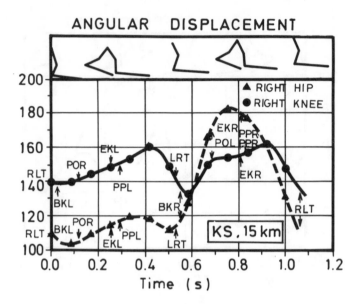

Figure 6—Relative angular displacement of hip and knee joint during one complete stride (two steps). Skier KS. See Figure 2 for symbols.

during leg push occurs when the velocity becomes positive.

MP commences hip extension about 0.1 sec. prior to knee extension (Figure 7) while KS begins about 0.08 sec. before knee extension. Both show a rapid knee flexion just prior to knee extension peaking at about −4 to −5 rad/s. Peak knee extension velocities were about 6 and 4 rad/s for MP and KS, respectively. Hip extension velocity peaks were about 9 and 8 rad/s for MP and KS, respectively. These extensions were preceded by a flexion at a peak velocity of about −2 rad/s for both skiers.

On average, for the five skiers, the peak knee extension velocity during push was 4.7 rad/s and the peak hip extension velocity was 8.7 rad/s. Overlays of the hip joint angular velocities show rather similar patterns for the five skiers (Figure 9). But knee joint angular velocity profiles showed a large degree of variability in both amplitude and phase between subjects.

Discussion

Dillman (1979) has presented some data which showed an average horizontal velocity of 4.64 m/s produced by a stride length of 2.88 m and a step rate of 1.61 steps/s. He makes the point that increases in velocity are accomplished more by increasing the step length than by increasing

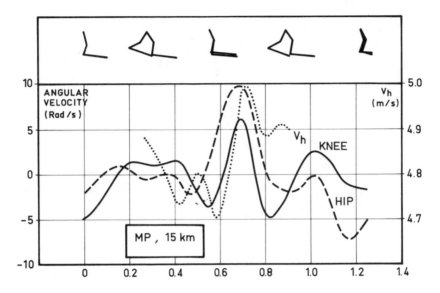

Figure 7—Relative angular velocity of hip and knee joint during one complete stride (two steps), and horizontal velocity (V_h) of the body center of gravity during the middle of the stride. Skier MP.

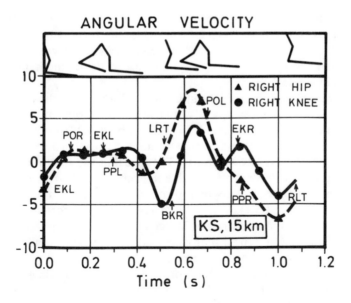

Figure 8—Relative angular velocity (rad/s) of hip and knee joint during one complete stride (two steps). Skier KS. See Figure 2 for symbols.

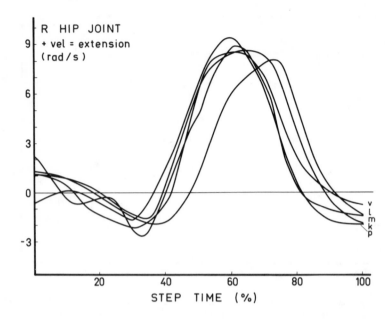

Figure 9—Relative angular velocity of the hip joint of five skiers normalized to percentage of single step time (from EKL to EKR; Figures 6 and 7 for example).

the step rate.

Our data would concur, in part, in that our average horizontal velocity of 4.81 m/s was achieved by a 2.96 m stride length and 1.63 step/s stride rate (Table 2). That is to say, a 3.7% increase in velocity over that shown by Dillman was produced by a 2.8% increase in stride length and a 0.6% increase in stride rate.

If, however, one observes the individual values among those of the five skiers presented, for example PV and KS at this point in the race, the conclusion is a little different. KS is skiing about 3.2% faster than skier PV, yet he has exactly the same step length (2.8 m) and a 3.6% faster step rate (1.75 steps/s vs. 1.69 steps/s). The fact that the fractional percentages do not total 100% is attributable to experimental error, probably in measurement of the step length and round-off error. Comparison of JL and PV shows that PV is skiing a bit faster but with a shorter step length.

Gagnon (1980) showed rather larger horizontal velocity fluctuations during a step (3.0-6.0 m/s) than occurred with the skiers in the present study (4.45-4.9 m/s). The skier used as an example from Gagnon's study was skiing at an average velocity of 5.74 m/s, but our skier, for comparison, was skiing at 4.70 m/s. It is possible that the velocity difference could account for the discrepancy. More likely, however, it is a difference created by the way the data were preprocessed. Because of high "noise" content in our data, obtained during competitive conditions, we were obliged to filter the coordinate values quite heavily (cf. Pezzack et al., 1977). This could have smoothed our curves somewhat more than that presented by Gagnon.

In conclusion, it appears that world class skiers achieve their speed in the diagonal technique in different ways. The horizontal velocity of the total body center of gravity profiles is similar in some ways but different in others. Angular displacement/time curves also show similarities across the five skiers but differences in detail, particularly during leg push. Hip joint angular velocity curves are very similar, but knee joint curves are peculiar to the individual.

Certainly, these highly skilled skiers are all exploiting basic biomechanical principles of propulsion, but further insight into precise mechanisms will have to await analysis of other joints such as the shoulder, elbow, wrist, and ankle. Definitive answers in propulsive mechanisms concerning between subject and within subject variability may not emerge until data from instrumented skis and poles are presented. In this study, only one step out of the thousands that are taken in a race was analyzed. Qualitatively, the step analyzed did not appear "atypical" to experienced coaches who observed the film. Much more data are required, however.

References

Dillman, C.J. 1979. Biomechanical determinations of effective cross-country skiing techniques. *J. of the United States Ski Coaches Association*, pp. 38-42.

Gagnon, M. 1980. Characteristics dynamics du pas alternatif en ski de fond. *Canadian Journal of Applied Sport Sciences* (in press).

Mietk, P., Hoessli, G., and Brenner, Y. 1978. *Skilanglauf.* (Cross-country Skiing.) Thesis in biomechanics, ETH Zurich, Switzerland.

Miller, D.I., and Nelson, R.C. 1973. *Biomechanics of Sport.* Lea and Febiger, Philadelphia.

Pezzack, J.C., Norman, R.W., and Winter, D.A. 1977. An assessment of derivative determining techniques used for motion analysis. *J. of Biomechanics* **10**:377-382.

Winter, D.A., Sidwall, H.G., and Hobson, D.A. 1974. Measurement and reduction of noise in kinematics of locomotion. *J. of Biomechanics* **7**:157-159.

Investigation of the Consistency of Movements
of Elite Judo Athletes

Tadeusz Bober, Alicja Rutkowska-Kucharska, and **Kornelia Kulig**
Academy of Physical Education, Wroclaw, Poland

Consistency of the disturbed movement with respect to the one programmed depends on the efficiency with which information is retrieved and transformed as well as on the magnitude of stimuli and synchronization of muscular tensions. Such movement is coordinated due to a flow of signals reaching two separate control "rings" (Chkhaidze, 1973).

Because the signals need about 0.12 sec. to travel the distance from the receptor to the effector, only movements lasting more than 0.2 sec. can be consciously controlled. Many movement tasks in sports last long enough ($t > 0.3$ sec.) to permit correction of errors (Bernstein, 1975; Morecki et al., 1971). Techniques used in a judo contest fall into this category. In judo, performance of the techniques is constantly disturbed by the opponent. Each of the contestants, while planning his actions, has to take into account the opponent's mass, speed, and direction of motion. During the workout, the judo athlete learns particular techniques by repeating them many times, very often with the same partner. In such a case, performance becomes optimal and schematic. At present the quality criteria for optimization of performance are unknown. It is believed that the following factors are involved (Gawronski, 1970): (a) precision—in the sense of the accuracy of reaching a determined position or the path; (b) speed in achieving a given position or trajectory, and (c) minimum of energy spent on the movement.

In the case of top athletes with good developmental adaptation to physical effort, the neuromuscular coordination which mainly affects the movement technique has a great influence on sport result (Kozlowski, 1978). It is thought that this process includes factors a and b. Moreover, the essence of the judo match consists of applying the learned technique under constantly changing conditions (unknown opponent, changing situation on the mat). For this reason, it was agreed that testing the accuracy and speed of the movement disturbed by external forces may have some cognitive and practical meaning for the testing of the judo athletes, and consequently, for programming training routines.

This objective was based on the assumption that the ability to create consistency of movements is desirable from the standpoint of judo athletes.

Procedure

In order to test the accordance of the executed movement with the programmed one, an electronic indicator of the error of movement, MURP[1], was used. The device consists of the following parts: an operational panel, a counter unit, a supply unit, and a slider with an indicator. The essential feature of the device is a set of electromagnets exerting forces which disturb the course of the movement performed by the subject (Bober and Szyslak, 1977). The operational panel includes the area with a drawn path programming the motion of the slider and four electromagnets affixed to the plate, which is able to rotate under the panel's lid.

The subject was required to lead the slider so that the tip of the indicator traveled precisely along the path. The task was performed with the upper extremity while in a standing position.

The motion of the slider was disturbed by the magnetic field of controlled intensity generated by the electromagnets. Evaluation of the test was based on the readings of the counters as follows: time of movement (sec.), off-the-path time (1 sec.), number of deviations from the path, the error factor proportional to the time of the error, and the distance of the indicators tip from the path. Each of the subjects was acquainted with the device and the method. Each test consisted of five trials, preceded by two "dry" runs.

The tests were performed by 61 judo athletes [31 seniors who were members of the national team (JS), plus 30 juniors (JJ), and 30 students of physical education (S)].

Results

The investigations included three consecutive experiments. The first experiment consisted of evaluation of the groups with respect to the level

---

[1]Application No. 92/2/79 has been submitted to the Polish Patent Office.

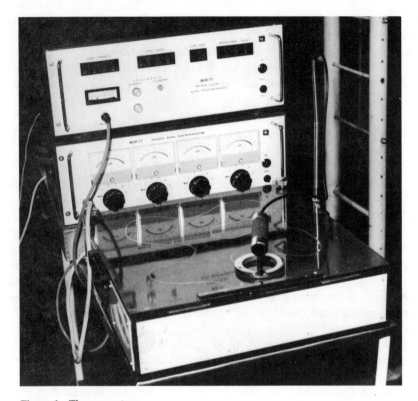

Figure 1—The apparatus.

of consistency of movement abilities (Table 1). The subject was required to perform the test as quickly and as accurately as possible, which means that the two features were equally important.

The revealed differences (statistically significant on the basis of *t*-test) among the groups of subjects, except in two cases, were not equivalent in interpretation (Table 2). The senior judo athletes achieved better results than the juniors, but comparison performed for these two groups and the control group (students) showed that the latter subjects completed the test differently. The students performed the task faster but less accurately. Similar results were obtained by Bober and Szyslak (1979).

The recorded difference in the way the test was performed led to the second experiment, which measured the time alotted for a single trial. In this test, a metronome was used to control the speed of tracing the determined sections of the path. This experiment involved a group of judo athletes (JS) and students (S).

The time recorded for the students in the first experiment was imposed on the senior judo athletes and vice versa. The results shown in Table 3

Table 1—Means and Standard Deviations of Four Parameters
of the Test Performed "Fast and Faultlessly"

Group	N	Time of trial(s)	Off-the-path time(s)	Number of deviations	Error factor
JS	31	36.0 ± 10.5	1.6 ± 1.5	6 ± 4.7	222 ± 223
JJ	30	39.6 ± 15.9	3.3 ± 2.5	10 ± 6.8	526 ± 402
S	30	25.8 ± 7.5	10.0 ± 4.1	24 ± 5.47	1539 ± 752.9

Table 2—t Values of the Differences Between Tested Groups

Parameters	JS-S	t JS-JJ	JJ-S
Time of trial	4.16[a]	1.00	4.45[a]
Off-the-path time	10.24[a]	3.09[a]	7.97[a]
Number of deviations	14.50[a]	2.53	9.79[a]
Error factor	8.88[a]	3.49[a]	6.74[a]

Note. [a]Statistically significant at 1% level of confidence.

indicate that shortening this time for the judo athletes deteriorated the accuracy of their movements, but a longer time for the students resulted in improvement in their precision; however, taking into account all factors pertaining to accuracy, the judo athletes achieved better results than the students, which was verified by the t-test. The calculated differences were statistically significant for 0.01 level of confidence for the time of the trial, the number of deviations, and the error factor; and the t values were, respectively, 8.48, 6.17, and 7.93.

The third experiment involved 10 (but very efficient) persons and consisted of repeating the trials many times. On two of them, the electrical activity (EMG) of selected muscles (biceps brachii, triceps brachii, latissimus dorsi, pectoralis major, extensor carpi radialis longus, flexor carpi radialis, extensor carpi ulnaris, and flexor carpi ulnaris) was simultaneously recorded. Assuming that the test reflects to some extent the consistency of movements with respect to a programmed movement (in spite of continuous disturbances), an attempt was made to find out whether this ability could be learned, especially during sport training.

To answer this question fully would require a longitudinal study on the group of subjects starting from the moment of their first judo workout;

Table 3—Means and Standard Deviations of Three Parameters
of the Test Performed "Faultlessly and Within the Time Limit"

Group	N	Time of trial(s)	Off-the-path time(s)	Number of deviations	Error factor
JS	31	26.6	2.4 ± 1.27	7 ± 5.57	532 ± 387
S	30	35.2	6.2 ± 3.7	11 ± 4.41	1499 ± 1017

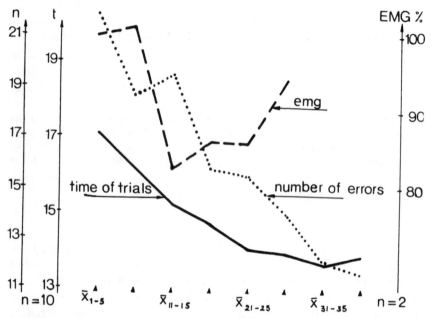

Figure 2—Results of time of trial, number of deviations, and electrical activity of muscles of 40 repetitions, grouped in means of five successive trials.

however, some evidence may be obtained from the results shown in Figure 2. The diagram presents the average results for each of five subsequent trials. The subjects constantly improved the time of the trial and reduced (or kept at a constant level) the number of errors. A large increase in the velocity of movement while maintaining the same number of errors could be achieved by a greater engagement of the muscles of the upper extremity holding and moving the indicator. It can be seen that the sum of average potentials recorded for eight muscles (and corresponding to the same seven points of the path) improved after 10 trials; thereafter, it levelled off and decreased in the last series of trials, probably due to fatigue. Taking these two factors into consideration, i.e., the test and the EMG, one may draw the conclusion that the response movement to the external disturbance and the consistency of movement with respect to the programmed movement can be improved by repeated exercises.

Discussion

In general, a negative relationship exists between the time of movement and the parameters characterizing the accuracy. Faster test performance is associated with less accuracy (Szyslak, 1978). This relation was observed in the present study, both for the students and for the members of the national team. For the latter group, the coefficients of correlation between the time of trial and the accuracy parameters were as follows: off-the-path time, ($r = -0.77$), number of deviations ($r = -0.60$), and error factor ($r = -0.56$).

These observations are in agreement with the hypothesis that the product of time and accuracy is constant. This means that shortening the time of the trial leads to deterioration of accuracy. It needs to be emphasized that, with respect to magnitude and direction, the specific character of the test consists of overcoming different, external forces. For this reason, the trial engages receptors to a greater extent than can be observed in other tests used in experimental psychology. The idea of the apparatus and the form of assignment given in the first experiment (to perform the test as fast and accurately as possible) was based on the assumption that the most efficient competitor surprises his opponent with quick actions executed in accordance with the pattern, regardless of the disturbance provided by the opponent. It is interesting to note that the judo athletes emphasized accuracy more than time as compared with the group of students. The second experiment, however, confirmed the hypothesis that the athletes performed the test not only in a different way but also with greater consistency of movement than persons not engaged in sport. This particular feature is probably associated with efficiency of the receptors, with speed of conducting the stimuli, and with better coordination of muscular forces (Szyslak, 1978). Although there are no reasons to reject the existence of the inherent predispositions which could affect the selection of sportsmen, it is justified to conclude on the basis of the results obtained from the first and the third experiments that this feature can be trained.

This observation may find practical implications in programming training routines whose purpose is to develop this feature much faster.

References

Bernstein, N.A. 1975. *Bewegungsphysiologie.* (Physiology of Movement.) Johann Ambrosius Barth, Leipzig.

Bober, T., and Szyslak, W. 1977. Measuring the adaptation of movement to outside forces. *Research Quarterly* **48**:800-804.

Bober, T., and Szyslak, W. 1979. Proba testowania dokladnosci ruchu zaklocanego silami zewnetrznymi u zawodnikow judo. (Testing of the precision of movement disturbed by outside forces in judo athletes.) *Wych. Fiz. i Sport,* (in press).

Chkhaidze, L.W. 1973. Biomechanics as the science of the coordination of the movements of man. In: Cirquilini, Venerando, and Wartenweiler (eds.), *Biomechanics III*, pp. 120-123. S. Karger, Basel, Switzerland.

Gawronski, R. 1970. *Bionika. System nerwowy jako uklad sterowania.* (Bionics. Nervous system as controlling one), pp. 469-475. PWN Warsaw.

Kozlowski, S.T. 1978. Wylonily sie nowe problemy z poznania funkcji organizmu podczas wysilku fizycznego . . . (New problems appeared while investigating the function of the human body during physical activity . . .) *Sport Wyczynowy* **2**:59-63.

Morecki, A., Ekiel, J., and Fidelus, K. 1971. Bionika ruchu. (Bionics of motion.) *Rozdial* **6**, pp. 307-352. PWN Warsaw.

Szyslak, W. 1978. Zdolnosc adaptacyjna ruchow czlowieka do zmieniajacych sie sil zewnetrznych. (The Adaptation of Human Motions to Changeable Outside Forces). Ph.D. dissertation, AWF, Wroclaw.

Immediate and Training Effects of Endurance-Type Exercise

Effect of Long Term Skiing on
Maximal and Submaximal Exercise Performance

Dag Linnarsson and **Brita Eklund**
Karolinska Institute and
Karolinska Hospital, Stockholm, Sweden

Fatigue after prolonged, severe exercise is a well-known phenomenon. Its physiological background, however, is not fully understood. In the present study, nonsteady state measurements of gas exchange during submaximal and maximal work were performed before and after a ski marathon. The main objective of the study was to investigate whether postexertional fatigue is accompanied by a decreased aerobic capacity, and if so, whether this in turn is caused by a failure to accelerate the O_2 transport.

Subjects and Methods

Eighteen of the participants in a 85.8 km ski marathon (Vasaloppet, Mora, Sweden) volunteered to take part in the study. All subjects were male. Age, height, and weight of the subjects ranged from 21-66 years, 1.69-1.87 m, and 56-90 kg, respectively.

Each subject was tested on two occasions, on the day before the race and within 1 hr. upon completion of the race. Like all other participants of the race, the subjects had free access to fluid and carbohydrates during the marathon. The testing procedure included submaximal and maximal exercise on a mechanically braked bicycle ergometer (Monark, Sweden). Work loads were selected to require 70 and 110% of the prerun maximal oxygen uptake. The subjects first performed submaximal exercise for 6 min. immediately followed by maximal exercise until exhaustion. Heart rate (HR) was obtained from chest (ECG) leads and a cardiotachometer. Gas exchange was measured continuously using a low resistance circuit (shown in Figure 1), where expired gases were con-

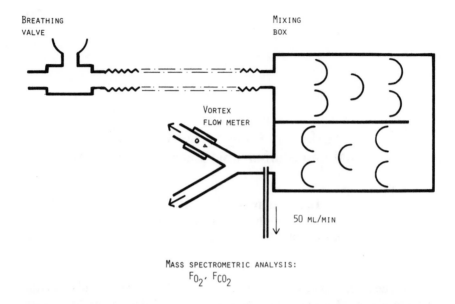

BREATHING
VALVE

MIXING
BOX

VORTEX
FLOW METER

50 ML/MIN

MASS SPECTROMETRIC ANALYSIS:
F_{O_2}, F_{CO_2}

Figure 1—Gas exchange measuring circuit, including low-resistance breathing valve, wide-bore respiratory tubing (I.D. 40 mm, volume 1 l), mixing box (volume 5 l) with hemicylindrical baffles to promote mixing, and flow meter.

tinuously mixed and then analyzed with a mass spectrometer (Centronic 200 MGA). Expired flow was measured by a vortex-type flow meter (Technitron, UK, type 3156). To reduce the resistance of the circuit, only half of the flow went through the vortex meter (I.D. 19 mm), the other half passing through a parallel tube of identical dimensions. The output of the flow meter was electronically damped (T = 14 sec.) to obtain ventilation ($\dot{V}_E$). Gas concentration signals from the mass spectrometer were recorded on a multichannel FM tape recorder, together with $\dot{V}_E$ and HR signals, for subsequent computations and presentation on a HP 9830 A computer with a HP 9866 plotter. Standard equations were used to compute oxygen uptake ($\dot{V}_{O_2}$), carbon dioxide elimination ($\dot{V}_{CO_2}$), and respiratory exchange ratio (R), with a sampling interval of 4 sec. The mean response time of the mixing box-analysator system depended on the ventilation (box volume/mean flow) and amounted to 6 and 3 sec., respectively, at ventilations of 60 and 120 $1 \cdot \min^{-1}$. Compared with the dynamics of the variables under study, the recording system was considered sufficiently fast-responding (Linnarsson, 1974).

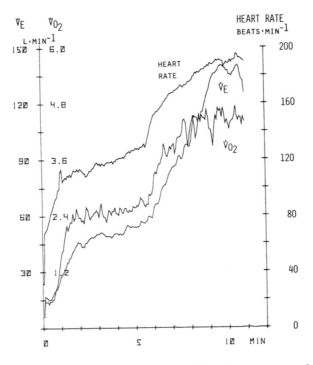

Figure 2—Original computer-generated plot of O_2 uptake ($\dot{V}_{O_2}$), ventilation ($\dot{V}_E$), and heart rate as a function of time during submaximal and maximal exercise in subject V.A. (control). Onset of maximal work is shown by the sudden secondary increase in HR.

Results

A typical recording showing the time courses of HR, $\dot{V}_{O_2}$ and $\dot{V}_E$ during submaximal and maximal work is shown in Figure 2. Values in the text and in Figures 3-5 refer to the final 30 sec. of each work period. During submaximal work, values for $\dot{V}_{O_2}$, HR, and $\dot{V}_E$ did not differ significantly between the tests before and after the race (Figures 3-5). The respiratory exchange ratio, however, was significantly reduced ($p < 0.01$) from 0.91 to 0.83. Maximal O_2 uptake averaged 4.04 1 · min^{-1} before the race and was significantly reduced ($p < 0.01$) to 90% of prerun control after the ski marathon (Figure 3). The decrease of $\dot{V}_{O_2}$ max showed a significant correlation ($p < 0.05$) with the average skiing speed during the intervening race.

Peak ventilation (Figure 4) and peak heart rate (Figure 5) were also significantly lower ($p < 0.01$) during postrun maximal exercise. At the same time, a given supramaximal work load could be sustained only 1.9 min. compared with 4.7 min. during prerun control.

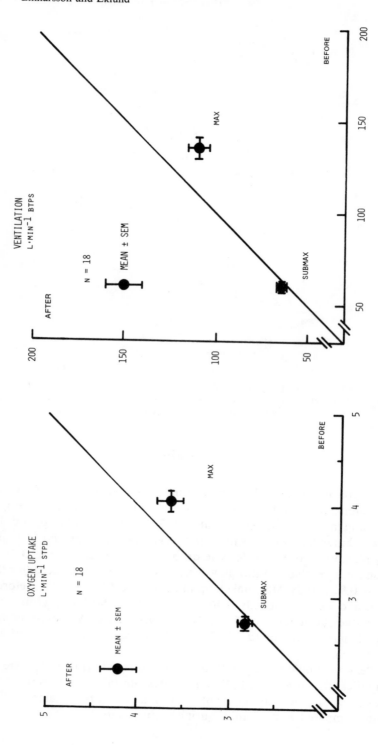

Figure 3—See text for Figure 5.

Figure 4—See text for Figure 5.

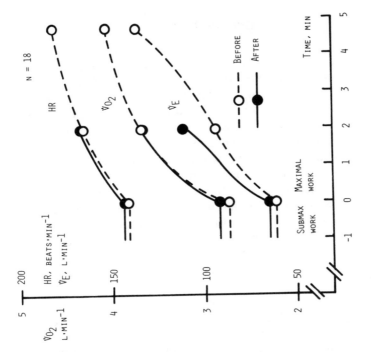

Figure 6—Oxygen uptake, $\dot{V}_E$, and HR as a function of time. Final values are shown for submaximal and maximal work as well as mean values for all individuals during the prerun maximal test at the time they interrupted the postrun maximal test.

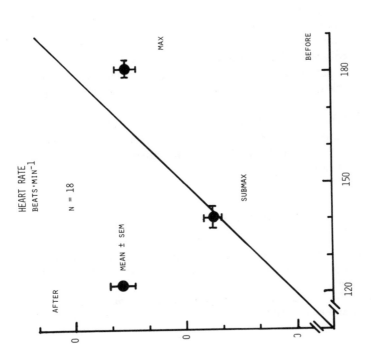

Figure 5—Postrun values for $\dot{V}_O$, $\dot{V}_E$, and HR during the last 30 sec. of submaximal and maximal exercise as a function of prerun control. Line of identity is also shown.

Discussion

Submaximal exercise performance was not greatly altered by prolonged exercise, but despite carbohydrate supply ad libitum during the race, the subjects' lowered R values after the race indicate a decreased utilization of carbohydrates and an increased utilization of lipids. This drop in R during submaximal exercise can be observed also as late as 24 hr. after prolonged, severe exercise and does not necessarily imply a complete glycogen depletion in the working muscles (Costill, 1973).

The lowered $\dot{V}_{O_2}$ max after prolonged severe exercise agrees well with the subjective experience of fatigue after the race. This deterioration of the maximal exercise performance can theoretically be caused by either a slowed acceleration of the O_2 transport or a decreased ability to supply energy anaerobically long enough to allow $\dot{V}_{O_2}$ to rise to its potential maximum level. The time course of $\dot{V}_{O_2}$ and the various processes involved in the O_2 transport (such as $\dot{V}_E$ and HR) should be slowed in the former case.

A comparison between $\dot{V}_{O_2}$, HR, and $\dot{V}_E$ during maximal work has therefore been made for each individual subject between the final values after the race and after the *same duration* of maximal work before the race (Figure 6). This comparison shows almost identical HR and $\dot{V}_{O_2}$ values, whereas $\dot{V}_E$ was 20% larger after the marathon. The present data therefore do not support the notion that the acceleration of the O_2 transport to its maximal rate is slowed after prolonged severe exercise. It is interesting that the subjects who performed best during the marathon, and who supposedly were the most well-trained and well-motivated subjects, also had the largest $\dot{V}_{O_2}$ reduction after the race. This observation speaks against lack of motivation as a cause for the postrun $\dot{V}_{O_2}$ max reduction.

It is concluded that decreased maximal aerobic power after prolonged severe exercise is due to factors—probably intramuscular—which cause exhaustion before the normally accelerating O_2 transport has reached its potential maximal rate.

References

Costill, D.L. 1973. Carbohydrate and lipid metabolism during successive days of prolonged running. In: V. Seliger (ed.) *Physical Fitness*, pp. 123-126. Karlova University, Prague.
Linnarsson, D. 1974. Dynamics of pulmonary gas exchange and heart rate changes at start and end of exercise. *Acta Physiol. Scand.*, Suppl. **415**.

Effects of Prolonged Cross-Country Skiing on Neuromuscular Performance

Jukka T. Viitasalo and **Paavo V. Komi**
Jyväskylä, Finland

Ira Jacobs and **Jan Karlsson**
Karolinska Institute, Stockholm, Sweden

Fatigue of the neuromuscular system during high-intensity exercise of a duration of 10-30 min. has been extensively studied. Few studies have examined the effects of several hours of exercise on the contractile characteristics of muscles in man. During extremely long cross-country ski races such as the Wasa, Finlandia, and Marcia Longa competitions, the participants exercise from 4-10 hr. at a high level of intensity. Thus, such a ski race offers an experimental model to investigate the effects of prolonged exercise-induced fatigue on subsequent exercise performance in man.

This study was undertaken to investigate the effects of the 85 km long Wasa ski race on some neuromuscular variables measured during isometric and dynamic muscle contractions.

Methods

Out of the 11,984 participants in the 1979 Wasa ski race (85 km), 23 skiers volunteered as subjects (Table 1). The subjects underwent a large test battery including: anthropometric measurement, muscle fiber typing, and the force production and relaxation phases of muscle contraction, including EMG variables. These variables were measured 1 day before and immediately after the race. The right m. vastus lateralis was biopsied using the percutaneous needle biopsy technique according to Bergstrom et al. (1962). Muscle fiber type distribution was calculated based upon myosin ATPase stainings (Padykula and Herman, 1955),

Table 1—Distribution of Anthropometric Measurements
and Skiing Time of Group

Group Characteristics	Range	X̄	SD
Age, years	21-66	36.1	12.1
Weight, kg	56.1-90.6	73.3	7.9
Height, cm	165-190	179.5	6.8
Percentage of FT	17.3-76.1	51.6	15.6
Percentage of FT area	17.9-77.3	53.8	17.0
Skiing time, hr.	5.37-9.49	7.94	1.53

Note. n = 23

and fiber areas were determined using a NADH tetrazolium reductase staining (Novikoff et al., 1961) and a method described by Tesch (1980).

Muscle contractile characteristics were measured using an identical protocol both the day before and 1-2 hr. after the race was finished on a Cybex (Lumex®, New York) dynamometer. After a few warm-up contractions, subjects were instructed to maximally extend the right leg and the torque produced was recorded on magnetic tape (Racal Store-7 tape recorder). The angular velocity of contraction was set and maintained at $180° \times s^{-1}$. Subsequently, upon presentation of simultaneous auditory and light signals, 10 maximal isometric knee extensions were performed at a knee angle of 120°. Subjects were instructed to extend the leg as quickly and as forcefully as possible upon presentation of the signals, to maintain the maximal contraction as long as the signals were activated (2.5 sec.), and to relax the muscles completely immediately after the disappearance of the signals. EMG was recorded bipolarly from m. rectus femoris, vastus lateralis, and vastus medialis during each contraction, using miniature size skin electrodes (Beckman) fixed to the middle part of each muscle belly. The recording points were carefully marked to ensure exactly the same placement of electrodes in pre and post measurements. The EMG signals (Brookdeal 9432 preamplifiers; 60 dB, 1 Hz-1kHz) were also stored on magnetic tape for subsequent analysis with an HP-21-MX computer. Isometric force time curves were further analyzed with regard to the force production and relaxation phases by calculating the highest value of slope coefficients, using 5 ms increments (for more detail, see Viitasalo et al., 1980). These variables are referred to as maximal rate of force development (RFD) and maximal rate of relaxation (RR).

Reaction times were also calculated and determined as the time begin-

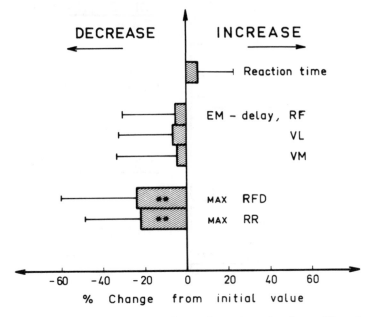

Figure 1—The effects of the prolonged skiing on the total reaction time and its motor time (= electromechanical delay, EM-delay), and on isometric force production (RFD) and relaxation (RR). **$p < .01$.

ning when the signals were activated to begin the isometric contractions and ending when force production reached the level of 5N. The total reaction time (TRT) was fractionated into its premotor (PMT) and motor time (MT) components by the onset of EMG activity according to Weiss (1965). The threshold for EMG was chosen separately for each reaction as described elsewhere (Viitasalo et al., 1980).

EMGs of the three muscles were analyzed for their integrals (IEMG) and mean power frequencies (MPF) of the power spectral density functions (PSDF) for the isometric and concentric contractions. The 2-sec. period at maximal force level was analyzed for the isometric contractions, and the 100 ms period in the middle part of the movement was analyzed for the dynamic contractions. The EMG analyzing methods have been described in more detail in a previous article (Viitasalo and Komi, 1975).

Conventional statistical methods, including the mean, standard deviation, standard error, coefficient of correlation, and the Student t-test, were used to analyze the results.

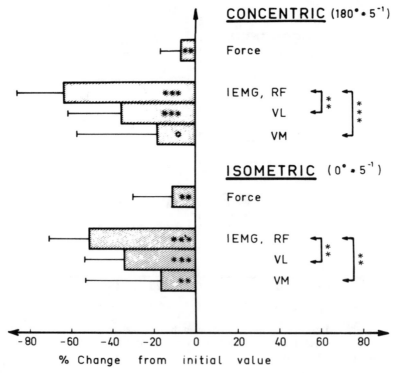

Figure 2—The effects of the ski race on maximal dynamic and isometric forces and IEMG integrals. RF = m. rectus femoris, VL = m. vastus lateralis, VM = m. vastus medialis. $°p < .1$, $**p < .01$, $***p < .001$.

Results

The effects of prolonged skiing were analyzed by calculating the percentage of change of each variable for each subject. The total reaction time with its premotor and motor components did not change significantly as shown in Figure 1. Yet the RFD and RR decreased significantly after the ski race (22% and 23%, respectively), suggesting that muscle tension was more slowly developed and relaxation was less efficient. Figure 2 summarizes the effects of the ski race on maximal isometric force and dynamic torque as well as on the IEMG results. These variables showed a significant decrease in both types of muscular contractions (10% and 7%, respectively). In addition, the IEMG of the m. rectus femoris decreased significantly more after prolonged skiing than did that of the m. vastus lateralis and m. vastus medialis. MPF of PSDF did not reveal any significant changes when the pre and postskiing values were compared. The percentage of change of each variable was correlated to the muscle fiber type distribution determined from the biopsy samples, and no significant correlation coefficient was found.

Discussion

The 85 km Wasa ski race induced no significant changes in reaction time or in its premotor or motor time components in the present study. An interpretation of this in accordance with previous findings (Karlsson, 1980) is that prolonged exercise-induced fatigue has no effect on the speed of the perceptual mechanisms involved in the initiation of muscular contraction. The most pronounced effects were found in relation to the rate of isometric force development and relaxation, maximal isometric and dynamic strength, and maximal integrated EMG measured during the maximal contractions.

The changes in RFD, RR, and maximal isometric force after prolonged exercise further supports an earlier study (Viitasalo and Komi, 1980). These changes may be a function of changes in the mechanograms of individual motor units, changes in their firing frequencies and/or in recruitment pattern. Studies where fatigue has been induced by exercise of a duration similar to that of the present study indicate that the force production and relaxation phases of the motor unit mechanograms become slower and maximal force decreases (Gydikov et al., 1976; Steg, 1964). A decrease in the firing frequencies of individual motor units has also been attributed to fatigue (Gydikov and Kosarov, 1973). These changes in the motor unit (MU) mechanograms and firing frequencies have been shown to be more marked in fast than in slow MUs (Gydikov et al., 1976; Gydikov and Kasarov, 1973; Steg, 1964). Moreover, the fatigue induced by high-intensity contractions has been thought to be due to the dropping out of primarily fast MUs (Gydikov et al., 1976). These factors, taken together with the findings of Viitasalo and Komi (1980), lead one to suspect a relationship between the extent of changes in RFD, RR, and maximal muscle force following prolonged skiing and skeletal muscle quality expressed as fiber type distribution. Such was not the case, however, in the present study. This may be directly due to differences in the metabolic status and concentrations of the precursors for muscle and blood lactate caused by the prolonged exercise. In the studies previously described, fatigue was induced by relatively short-term intense exercise, where the lactate accumulation was supposedly, or reported to be, elevated and thus pH decreased. Such a condition probably impairs the force production capabilities of the neuromuscular system as discussed in more detail by Karlsson (1980) and Viitasalo (1980).

After prolonged exercise of a 4-hr. duration, intramuscular glycogen stores are severely reduced and blood and muscle lactates lower than in control experiments when subsequent high-intensity exercise is performed (Jacobs, 1981; Karlsson, 1971). Thus, it seems reasonable to assume that the effects of prolonged exercise-induced fatigue could differ from those of short-term, high-intensity-induced fatigue on the basis of the ability to form lactate in two different situations. An assumed reduced lactate accumulation during the repeated isometric contractions following the ski race may also explain why the mean power frequency of the EMG power spectral density was not altered after prolonged exercise.

Even though no significant changes were found in reaction time or its components, the great decrease in electrical activity after skiing suggests reduced neural input to the muscle via alpha-motoneurons (central fatigue). The reduction of IEMG may also be due to failure in transmission of action potential through the neuromuscular junction or in its propagation along the muscle fibers. During short-term, intense exercise-induced fatigue, failure in neuromuscular transmission and in propagation of muscle action potential may not necessarily be a limiting factor (Asmussen and Mazin, 1978a, 1978b; Bigland-Ritchie et al., 1975). Thus, the weakening and slowing of the contractile mechanisms after prolonged exercise may be partly due to central fatigue which, according to Asmussen and Mazin (1978a, 1978b), may be affected by the balance between the outflow of inhibitory and facilitatory impulses from the periphery to the central nervous system.

The significantly greater reduction of IEMG activity in m. rectus femoris than in m. vastus lateralis or m. vastus medialis following skiing was one of the most obvious findings in the present study. This suggests that m. rectus femoris was more fatiguable due to either greater susceptibility or to more extensive activation during skiing than the vasti group. The former explanation is supported by the findings of Kwatny et al. (1970), which suggests that the m. rectus femoris is a faster muscle than the two other knee extensors studied. Fast muscles have been shown to be less resistant to fatigue than slow ones (Burke and Edgerton, 1975) and the contractile features of muscle rich in FT fibers to be more impaired than ST rich muscle when strength-type exercise is performed after prolonged exercise (Jacobs et al., 1981). The latter explanation is hypothetical and requires further empirical support, yet it is based upon the anatomically and functionally different behavior of the knee extensor muscles during skiing. The vasti group is a pure knee extensor, whereas m. rectus femoris, as a two-joint muscle, functions in both knee extension and hip flexion. In knee extension during the stance phase of skiing, we can assume that each of the quadriceps muscles is active. At least at the beginning of the swing phase, activation of the hip flexors is required. M. rectus femoris, as a hip flexor, might also be active during the swing phase, when the m. vastus lateralis and m. vastus medialis are probably silent. This explanation is in line with the results reported by Frigo et al. (1978), who studied the activity of the m. rectus femoris during running. Thus, according to this hypothesis, the m. rectus femoris is active far longer during skiing than its vasti counterparts and, therefore, is more fatigued as a result of the ski race.

Summary

After prolonged (5-9 hr.) skiing, maximal isometric and dynamic knee extension forces were significantly reduced, when compared to the before skiing values. It was also found that a significant slowing in the rate of isometric force production and relaxation occurred as well as a reduction in maximal myoelectrical activity of the three superficial knee extensor muscles. The reduction in IEMG of the m. rectus femoris was significantly greater than the IEMGs of the vastus lateralis and vastus medialis muscles.

References

Asmussen, E., and Mazin, B. 1978a. Recuperation after muscular fatigue by "diverting activities." *Eur. J. Appl. Physiol.* **38**:1-7.

Asmussen, E., and Mazin, B. 1978b. A central nervous component in local muscular fatigue. *Eur. J. Appl. Physiol.* **38**:9-15.

Bergstrom, J. 1962. Muscle electrolytes in man. *Scand. J. Clin. Lab. Invest.*, Suppl. **68**.

Bigland-Ritchie, B., Hosking, G.P., and Jones, D.A. 1975. The site of fatigue in sustained maximal contractions of the quadriceps muscle. *J. Physiol.* (London) **250**:45-46P.

Burke, R.E., and Edgerton, V.R. 1975. Motor unit properties and selective involvement in movement. In: J.H. Wilmore and J.F. Keogh (eds.), *Exercise and Sport Sciences Reviews*, Vol. 3, Franklin Institute Press, Philadelphia.

Frigo, C., Pedotti, A., and Santambrogio, G.C. 1978. A correlation between muscle length and EMG activity during running. *Int. Congress of Sports Sciences*, July 25-29, 1978, Edmonton, Canada.

Gydikov, A., Dimitrov, G., Kosarov, D., and Dimitrova, N. 1976. Functional differentiation of motor units in human opponens pollicis muscle. *Exp. Neurol.* **50**:36-57.

Gydikov, A., and Kosarov, D. 1973. Physiological characteristics of the tonic and phasic motor units in human muscles. In: A.A. Gydikov, N.T. Tankov, and D.S. Kosarov (eds.), *Motor control*, pp. 75-94. Plenum Press, NY.

Jacobs, I. 1981. Lactate concentrations after short, maximal exercise at various glycogen levels. *Acta Physiol. Scand.* **111**:465-469.

Jacobs, I., Kaiser, P., and Tesch, P. 1981. The effects of glycogen exhaustion on maximal, short time performance. (this volume).

Karlsson, J. 1971. Lactate and phosphagen concentrations in working muscle of man. *Acta Physiol. Scand.,* Suppl. **358**.

Karlsson, J. 1980. Localized muscular fatigue: Role of muscle metabolism and substrate depletion. In: R. Hutton and D. Miller (eds.), *Exercise and Sport Science Reviews,* Vol. 7, pp. 1-42. Franklin Institute Press, Philadelphia.

Kwatny, E., Thomas, D.H., and Kwatny, H.G. 1970. An application of signal processing techniques to the study of myoelectric signals. IEEE Transactions on Bio-Medical Engineering **17**(4):303-312.

Novikoff, A.B., Shin, W-Y., and Drucher, J. 1961. Mitochondrial localization of oxidative enzymes: staining results with two tetrazolium salts. *J. Biophys. Biochem. Cytol.* **9**:47-61.

Padykula, H.A., and Herman, E. 1955. The specificity of the histochemical method for adenosine triphosphatase. *J. Histochem. Cytochem.* **3**:170-195.

Steg, G. 1964. Efferent innervation and rigidity. *Acta Physiol. Scand.,* Suppl. **225**, p. 61.

Tesch, P. 1980. Muscle fatigue in man. With special reference to lactate accumulation during short-term intense exercise. *Acta Physiol. Scand., Suppl.* **480**.

Viitasalo, J. 1980. Neuromuscular performance in voluntary and reflex contraction with special reference to muscle structure and fatigue. *Studies in Sport, Physical Education and Health* **12**, University of Jyväskylä, Jyväskylä, Finland.

Viitasalo, J.T., and Komi, P.V. 1975. Signal characteristics of EMG with special reference to reproducibility of measurements. *Acta Physiol. Scand.* **93**:531-539.

Viitasalo, J.T., and Komi, P.V. 1981. Effects of fatigue on isometric force and relaxation-time characteristics in human muscle. *Acta Physiol. Scand.* **111**(1):87-95.

Viitasalo, J.T., Saukkonen, S., and Komi, P.V. 1980. Reproducibility of measurements of selected neuro-muscular performance variables in man. *Electromyogr. Clin. Neurophysiol.* **20**:487-501.

Weiss, A.D. 1965. The locus or reaction time change with set, motivation and age. *J. of Gerontology* **20**:60-64.

Metabolic and Hemodynamic Effects
of Physical Training in Middle-aged Men
—A Controlled Trial

**Esko Länsimies, Eino Hietanen, Jussi K. Huttunen, Osmo Hanninen,
Kati Kukkonen, Rainer Rauramaa, and Erkki Voutilainen**
University of Kuopio, Finland

Epidemiological studies have suggested that regular physical activity at work or during leisure time protects man against coronary heart disease (Morris et al., 1973; Paffenbarger and Hale, 1975). Final proof for this contention is, however, difficult to attain because of the problems associated with controlled exercise trials. On the other hand, indirect evidence for the beneficial effects of physical activity can be obtained from the studies concerning the effects of exercise on the risk factors of coronary heart disease like serum lipoproteins, glucose tolerance, and blood pressure.

A controlled trial was reported on the effects of mild to moderate physical exercise on serum lipids and lipoproteins (Huttunen et al.,1979). This article will describe changes exhibited in the metabolic and hemodynamic parameters of the previous study, before and after discontinuation of supervised training.

Methods

A detailed description of the study group and the design of the controlled part of the investigation has been published elsewhere (Huttunen et al., 1979). Briefly, 100 asymptomatic middle-aged men were randomly assigned to exercise and control groups after two baseline examinations carried out at a 2-month interval (time points I and II). Thereafter, the exercise group (Group A) participated in a 4-month supervised exercise program consisting of jogging, swimming, skiing, and cycling. The in-

tensity of training was adjusted so that the target heart rate during the
three to four weekly exercise sessions was resting heart rate +0.40 ×
(maximal heart rate - resting heart rate) during the first 2 months (i.e.,
between time points II and III) and resting heart rate + 0.66 (maximal
heart rate - resting heart rate) during the second 2 months of the training
(i.e., between time points III and IV). The subjects in the control group
(Group B) were asked to maintain their previous exercise habits during
this part of the study.

After the 4-month training period (i.e., after time point IV), participants of Group A were informed of the results of the training program. They were advised to continue their training as previously but
without supervision or further instructions. Subjects in Group B, who
had been inactive until this time point, were given an individualized (but
unsupervised) training program consisting of three 30-40 min. weekly
bouts of brisk walking. Final evaluation of the physical performance and
various metabolic and hemodynamic parameters was carried out in both
groups after 6 months of unsupervised training (time point V).

At each time point, a 12-hr. postabsorptive blood sample was drawn
for blood glucose and serum lipoprotein determinations. A progressive
submaximal exercise test was performed in the afternoon to determine
maximal oxygen uptake and the response of various hemodynamic parameters to exercise testing. The work load was increased stepwise in
four consecutive 3-min. periods to attain 85% of the age-specific maximal pulse level. Maximal oxygen uptake ($\dot{V}O_2$) was calculated using the
indirect method (Lange-Andersen et al., 1971). Plasma lipids and
lipoproteins were determined with the procedure recommended in Lipid
Research Clinic Manual of Laboratory Operations (1974). Statistical
significance was tested with a paired t-test.

Results

As shown in Table 1, a highly significant increase in maximal oxygen
uptake was observed in Group A during the period of supervised training
(between time points II and IV). Discontinuation of the exercise instructions did not impair the physical performance: $\dot{V}O_2$ was still significantly
elevated after 6 months of unsupervised training (time point V). In contrast, no change was seen in $\dot{V}O_2$ Group B between time points II and IV.
This was expected, because the participants of this group were requested
to maintain their previous exercise habits during this period. On the
other hand, a significant increase in oxygen uptake was observed in this
group between time points IV and V, i.e., during the training period consisting of regular brisk walking. Body mass index decreased slightly in

Table 1—The Effect of Training on Maximal Oxygen Uptake ($\dot{V}_{O_2}$) and Body Mass Index (BMI) in Groups A and B (Mean ± SE)

Physiological factor	Group	Time point II	Time point IV	Time point V
$\dot{V}_{O_2}$ (ml/kg·min)	A	42.4 ± 1.1	47.6 ± 1.0	46.7 ± 1.3
	B	43.9 ± 1.0	42.9 ± 1.0[a]	46.0 ± 1.0
BMI (kg/m²)	A	25.9 ± 0.4	25.5 ± 0.4	25.8 ± 0.4
	B	26.6 ± 0.4	26.4 ± 0.4	26.3 ± 0.4

[a]Significant difference between the groups = $p < 0.05$.

Table 2—The Effect of Training on Serum Lipids and Lipoproteins in Groups A and B (Mean ± SE)

Lipid fraction	Group	Time point II	Time point IV	Time point V
			mmol/l	
Cholesterol	A	6.70 ± 0.20	6.10 ± 0.10	6.10 ± 0.10
	B	6.80 ± 0.20	6.30 ± 0.20	6.40 ± 0.10
HDL cholesterol	A	1.27 ± 0.04	1.40 ± 0.05	1.36 ± 0.05
	B	1.24 ± 0.04	1.26 ± 0.03[a]	1.25 ± 0.04[a]
LDL cholesterol	A	4.74 ± 0.16	4.20 ± 0.13	4.11 ± 0.15
	B	4.82 ± 0.14	4.52 ± 0.15	4.38 ± 0.14
Triglycerides	A	1.52 ± 0.09	1.30 ± 0.08	1.13 ± 0.07
	B	1.43 ± 0.14	1.58 ± 0.13[a]	1.31 ± 0.07

[a]Significant difference between the groups = $p < 0.05$.

Group A between time points II and IV, but it returned to the original level during the unsupervised part of the training program. No changes were observed in Group B.

Total serum cholesterol (Table 2) decreased significantly in both groups during the controlled part of the study (between time points II and IV) and remained constant in both groups between time points IV and V. The changes in low-density lipoprotein (LDL) cholesterol were similar to those seen in total serum cholesterol. Total serum triglyceride and very low-density lipoprotein (VLDL) triglyceride concentration decreased significantly in Group A between time points II and IV. The change further increased during the period of unsupervised training. No

Table 3—The Effect of Training on Resting Heart Rate and
Heart Rate 15 Min. After Submaximal Exercise Test (Mean ± SE)

Heart rate (min⁻¹) and work load	Group	Time point II	Time point IV	Time point V
At rest	A	73 ± 2	72 ± 2	69 ± 2
	B	75 ± 1	77 ± 1[b]	74 ± 1[b]
After exercise	A	76 ± 1	76 ± 2	75 ± 1
	B	80 ± 1	85 ± 2[b]	77 ± 1
Work load (W)[a]	A	190 ± 4	223 ± 1	212 ± 1
	B	194 ± 4	208 ± 4	209 ± 1

Note. [a]At the end of the test.
[b]Significant difference between the groups = $p < 0.05$.

changes were seen in Group B before or during the exercise program.

The concentration of HDL cholesterol increased significantly in Group A between time points II and IV and decreased slightly after discontinuation of the supervised training. Despite the small reduction during the second part of the study, the level of HDL cholesterol was still significantly higher at the end of the investigation (time point V) than before the beginning of the training program. The level of HDL cholesterol remained constant in Group B throughout the study even though there was an increase in $\dot{V}_{O_2}$ between time points IV and V.

The effect of various modes of exercise training on resting and postexercise heart rates are shown in Table 3. The resting heart rate decreased slightly in Group A both during the period of supervised and the period of unsupervised training. A similar decrease was also seen in Group B during the walking program (i.e., between time points IV and V). The postexercise heart rate (recorded 15 min. after the submaximal test) remained unchanged in Group A, whereas in Group B, an increase was observed between time points II and IV and a decrease between time points IV and V. The changes in postexercise heart rate in Group B are, however, probably due to an inappropriately high work load (in relation to the physical condition) used in the exercise testing at time point IV (see Table 3).

The resting and postexercise blood pressure values recorded during the study are shown in Table 4. A parallel and highly significant decrease in the resting systolic pressure was seen in both groups. On the other hand, no change was seen in the resting diastolic pressure or in the postexercise systolic or diastolic pressure in either group.

Table 4—The Effect of Training on Systolic (SBP) and
Diastolic (DBP) Blood Pressure Recorded Before and
After Submaximal Exercise Test in Groups A and B (Mean ± SE)

Blood pressure	Group	Time point II	Time point IV	Time point V
			mmHg	
SBP				
At rest	A	130 ± 2	122 ± 2	123 ± 2
	B	128 ± 2	123 ± 2	123 ± 1
After exercise	A	123 ± 2	121 ± 2	122 ± 1
	B	124 ± 2	125 ± 2	125 ± 2
DBP				
At rest	A	84 ± 1	83 ± 1	84 ± 1
	B	84 ± 1	86 ± 1	86 ± 1
After exercise	A	84 ± 1	82 ± 1	84 ± 1
	B	86 ± 1	87 ± 1[a]	88 ± 1[a]

Note. Work loads at the end of the test are given in Table 3.
[a]Significant difference ($p < 0.05$) between the groups.

The mean arterial pressures (MAP) recorded during the exercise tests at the various time points are shown in Figures 1 and 2. Supervised training lowered MAP at low work loads (50-100 W) in Group A, whereas the response to the higher work loads remained unchanged. During the period of unmonitored training the entire curve shifted to the left. A reduction in MAP at low work loads but not at high work loads was seen in Group B after the period of walking exercises. No significant alterations in the response of the rate-pressure product (mmHg $\times$ min^{-1}) to various work loads were seen in either group during the study (data not shown).

Discussion

The controlled part of our study indicated that a supervised exercise program consisting of jogging and skiing with mild to moderate intensity lowers serum triglyceride levels and raises serum HDL level in previously inactive middle-aged men. The present report further demonstrates that these changes are not temporary: the changes in serum triglycerides and HDL cholesterol persisted during 6 months of unsupervised training. On the other hand, observations made of the participants in the walking pro-

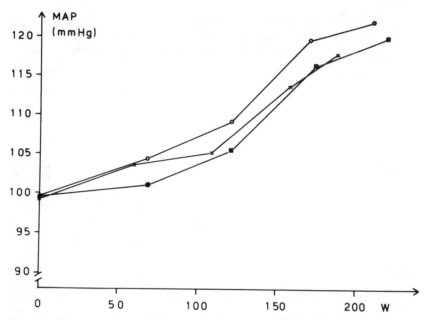

Figure 1—Effect of work load (W) on mean arterial pressure (MAP; mmHg) during submaximal exercise tests in Group A. X = Time point II (before the beginning of the exercise program).
■ = Time point IV (at the end of the supervised training program consisting of jogging and similar activity).
O = Time point V (at the end of the unsupervised part of the training program). Mean of 40-45 observations.

gram suggest that this type of exercise may not influence HDL cholesterol concentration; despite the increase in the oxygen uptake capacity. It remains to be shown whether the lack of change in HDL cholesterol under these conditions is due to the different quality or to the somewhat lower intensity of the walking program.

A small but significant reduction in the resting heart rate was seen in the participants both during the jogging and walking programs. This finding is in agreement with earlier reports on resting bradycardia in healthy young men after training programs of short duration and relatively low intensity (Frick et al., 1970).

Systolic blood pressure decreased significantly in the exercise group during the controlled part of our study; however, a parallel reduction was also seen in the control group, indicating that the change was due to the well-known placebo effect associated with repeated blood pressure measurements (Frick et al., 1963). It should be noted, on the other hand, that the response of the mean arterial pressure to low work loads (but not to high work loads) decreased significantly during both training pro-

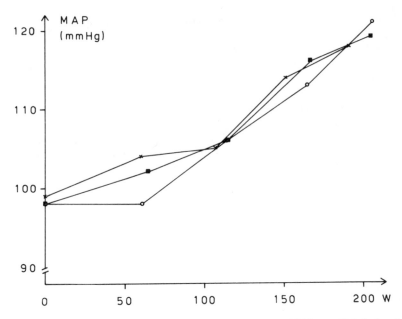

Figure 2—Effect of work load (W) on mean arterial pressure (MAP; mmHg) during the submaximal exercise tests in Group B. X = Time point II (before the beginning of the control period).
■ = Time point IV (at the end of the control period).
O = Time point V (at the end of the training program consisting of brisk walking).

grams, but not during the control period. Thus, it is likely that regular physical activity will lower the blood pressure response to mild and moderate physical activities associated with everyday life.

In summary, we conclude that moderate physical exercise consisting of jogging or similar activity will favorably influence several risk factors of coronary heart disease. Training programs composed of brisk walking alone may be less effective in this respect, although a significant increase in oxygen uptake is obviously attained also by this type of training.

References

Frick, M.H., Konttinen, A., and Sarajas, H.S.S. 1963. Effects of physical training on circulation at rest and during exercise. *Am. J. Cardiol.* **12**:142-147.

Frick, M.H., Sjogrén, A.-L., Perasalo, J., and Pajunen, S. 1970. Cardiovascular dimensions and moderate physical training in young men. *J. Appl. Physiol.* **29**:452-455.

Huttunen, J.K., Lansimies, E., Voutilainen, E., Ehnholm, C., Hietanen, E., Penttila, I., Siitonen, O., and Rauramaa, R. 1979. Effect of moderate physical exercise on serum lipoproteins. A controlled study with special reference to serum high-density lipoproteins. *Circulation* **60**:1220-1229.

Lange-Andersen, K., Shephard, R.J., Denoli, H., Varnauskas, E., and Masironi, R. 1971. *Fundamentals of exercise testing.* World Health Organization, Geneva.

Lipid Research Clinics Manual of Laboratory Operations (Vol.1). Lipid and Lipoproteins Analysis, HEW publication No. NIH 75-628. Washington DC, US Government Printing Office, 1974.

Morris, J.N., Chave, S.P., Adam, C., Sirey, C., Epstein, L., and Sheehan, D.J. 1973. Vigorous exercise in leisure-time and the incidence of coronary heart disease. *Lancet* **1**:333-339.

Paffenbarger, R.S., and Hale, W.E. 1975. Work activity and coronary heart mortality. *N. Engl. J. Med.* **292**:545-550

A Simple Method to Control Fatigue
in Endurance Training

Wojciech Czajkowski
Academy of Physical Education, Warsaw, Poland

During the many years as a physician for cross-country skiing teams, I have had the chance to work with the coaches in evaluating the working capacity and the fatigue level of the skiers. In order to estimate the influence of arduous endurance training upon the skiers, I was forced to carry out my observations either in the mountains or in the polar circle zone, without the help of a modern physiological laboratory. Thus, I have attempted to adapt the orthostatic test to the needs of evaluating the performance of the skier. It is known that as the consequence of overfatigue or overstrain, a disorder of a developing nervous system may possibly occur. This disorder can be studied with the orthostatic test. The first attempt was to evaluate the advantages and correct interpretation of this test when used as an estimation of the level of fatigue or for determination of the skier's performance level.

Methods

The orthostatic test was usually conducted in the morning, immediately after the skiers awoke. Initially, heart rate (HR) and blood pressure measurements were taken three times: (a) immediately after awakening, (b) after changing from the lying position to the standing position, and (c) after 60 sec. in the standing position. Immediately upon arising, HR was observed to increase by about 20 beats per min. However, within 15 to 20 sec., HR decreased, reaching a value only somewhat higher than that observed in the lying position. No change of HR was observed within the next minute. Thus, the decrease in HR was considered to be the most distinctive factor in evaluating the fatigue and working capacity of the skiers exposed to endurance training. Because the response of the blood pressure was usually nontypical, we decided to measure only HR. The following sequence was used in monitoring HR: (a) in the lying position and (b) 20 sec. after assuming the standing position, i.e., when the decrease of HR had occurred. When the initial HR measurement was low and the second recording was only 4-8 beats per min. higher than that of the first measurement, we considered the test result to be a good one.

Results and Interpretation

Our observations of 10 female cross-country skiers from the Polish National Team have been carried out during a period of almost 2 years. Depending on the contact frequency with skiers, the orthostatic test has been carried out two to three times per week, sometimes less frequently. When a test result was significantly different from the one obtained previously, the test was repeated over 3 consecutive days. These test results which were considered the most representative of any of the training periods were then compared with a real sport conditioning and working capacity level. The level of sport conditioning and working capacity was determined by the competition performance results as well as by the results obtained in periodical test runs during the summer and winter. Furthermore, we observed our skiers during their interval and strength training practice.

In nine cases, good correlation existed between the orthostatic test results and the sport conditioning and working capacity level. Only in one case was such a correlation not always observable. Figures 1 through 4 present the most representative examples. The exercise capabilities of the female skier in Figure 1 were observed during the entire summer of 1970 and confirmed by a complete set of physiological tests. The orthostatic test also gave good results during this summer period. In the latter part of September and in the beginning of October, the orthostatic test gave poor values. Nevertheless, we decided that she should continue her training because she felt good and her sport results in the periodical control tests were good too; however, within the next few weeks her sport performance decreased and finally her physical capacity decreased drastically. The orthostatic test results were also very poor at this time. At this point, she stopped training and underwent a medical examination. No pathological changes were revealed during the 2 weeks of medical observation. Thus, she returned gradually to physical activity, and in November, she started her regular training program again. At the beginning of her return, the training intensity level was kept low. When the orthostatic test results had changed for the better, the training became more intensive. During the winter season of 1971, this skier was

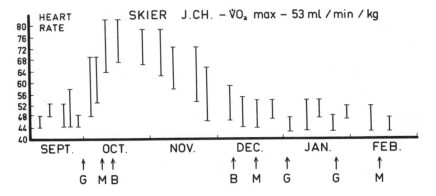

Figure 1—Orthostatic test results of female skier J.CH.

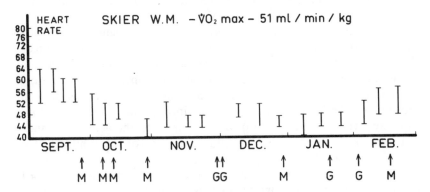

Figure 2—Orthostatic test results of female skier W.M.

able to reach a high level of working capacity and she achieved good results in competition.

From Figure 2, it may be noted that the orthostatic test results of this skier were predominantly good (i.e., the value of the initial pulse rate measurement was low, and the difference between the first and the second measurement was rather small). She was able to maintain her sport performance at a good level. Only at the beginning of the more intensive training period (September) were the orthostatic test results observed to decrease. Thus, some corrections of the training program were made. Afterwards, the test results improved and reached the normal level. The skier also performed well in competition.

The following year it was learned that this test was of little value for evaluations of the sport conditioning of our female skiers, because results showed a hyperexcitable reaction of their nervous systems during

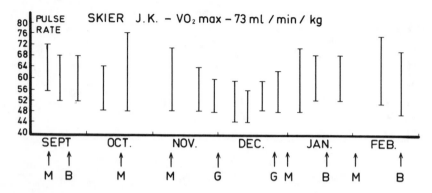

Figure 3—Orthostatic test results of male Nordic skier J.K. prior to 1976 Olympic Games.

the testing. This phenomenon occurred because all the skiers knew how noteworthy this examination was considered.

Thus, we started a similar experiment with a male team in Nordic competition. Not all skiers from this group were informed about the aim and the results of the testing. A good correlation between the orthostatic test results and the level of sport conditioning was observed in this group. Moreover, the competition performance result corresponded with the orthostatic test value. In order to get more information about the working capacity level, the maximum oxygen uptake and the acid-base balance test were investigated during the autumn (i.e., before beginning the hard training period).

Figure 3 shows the orthostatic test results of our best skier in Nordic competition before the Olympic Games in Innsbruck. It should be emphasized that this skier had an unstable type of nervous system reaction. The results of his competitive performance in the most important meets (such as the Olympic Games or the World Championship) were poor. He was, however, able to win several times in the less important meets and beat many champions. After a decrease in the working capacity level was observed in August and September, he was gradually exposed to the full intensity training program, and during this period, a good correlation between the orthostatic test values and the periodical efficiency test and competitive performance results were observed. During the competitive season, the orthostatic test results were poorer, with a concomitant decrease in the competition performance results.

In the following few years, the orthostatic test was carried out on a group of male national team cross-country skiers; however, in this experiment we decided to study the fatigue level alone, and no attempt was made to estimate the competitive performance of the skiers. In this group, the maximum oxygen uptake was determined twice a year. When the orthostatic test values changed for the worse, we were prepared to

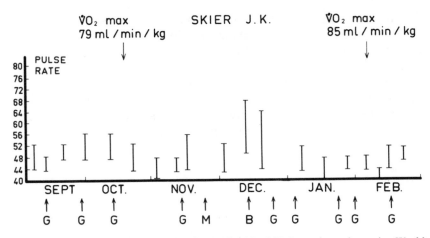

Figure 4—Orthostatic test results of male Nordic skier J.K. just prior to becoming World Champion in 1978.

make some corrections in the training program. These corrections referred mainly to a change of the duration of training, and only seldom in the level of intensity of training. For example, we let the skiers decrease the distance of cross-country hiking, but we had them increase the roller skiing distances or the training frequency to develop strength and jumping ability. In my opinion, this allowed our skiers to avoid symptoms of fatigue and overstrain.

Figure 4 presents results of our best skier for a few months before he became the World Champion in 1978. Despite the great intensity of training, good results in the orthostatic test were observed even during the high mountain training. The training there was very arduous but varied. When training in the polar circle zone, our test result was observed to decrease, and his competitive results in December were poor. The skier was then instructed to rest for a few days. As the orthostatic test results improved, normal training program was renewed. In January and February, good results of the orthostatic test corresponded with good competitive performances. A very good value on our test was observed during the training in Lahti, Finland, 2 weeks before the World Championships. During the competition, the orthostatic test results were, however, somewhat worse. This was due to emotional stress during the days of competition. His performances, however, were very good.

Conclusions

1. The orthostatic test presented is easy to carry out and interpret.

2. It is interesting that the value of this test can be observed to change before any decrease of the working capacity is noticed.

3. When a decrease in the orthostatic test result is observed, a change in training factors is recommended.

4. When a value of the orthostatic tests is really poor, and a large decrease in the working capacity occurs, a longer rest is recommended.

5. If one works with a person who has a hyperexcitable psychological reaction, it is difficult to interpret the orthostatic test results.

Evaluation of Physical Capacity
in Chilean Volleyball Players

Roberto M. Montecinos, Jose E. Guajardo,
Luis Lara, Francisco Jara, and Patricio Gatica
Pontificia Universidad Catolica de Chile, Talca, Chile

The group of factors mentioned by Astrand (1970) that determine physical capacity are characteristics which can change, and therefore modify, athletic capacity in individuals. Those variables which change, and which alter such athletic capacity can be measured using proven methods.

Several publications have dealt with physical capacity and athletic improvement, and they have contributed to an understanding of the modification of physical capacity in athletes in general (Astrand, 1976; Dal Monte, 1979; Donoso et al., 1977); however, data on volleyball players are scarce, and those which exist correspond to populations with homogeneous biotypological characteristics from developed countries. Such is not the case with the Chilean athletic population, which comes from diverse ethnic groups and socioeconomic levels. For this reason, we were interested in applying a series of feasible techniques to a group of Chilean volleyball players and in relating the results to those obtained in similar studies in other countries.

The evaluation of the practice of volleyball has shown that the better trained teams are those which, together with improvement of technique, have introduced speed and strength into their training programs. This supports Dal Monte's (1979) modern classification of the sport as aerobic-anaerobic and explains the level of importance which physical preparation has acquired in modern volleyball. This study was designed to help establish reference values for functional and anatomical characteristics of Chilean players of different age, sex, and technical level.

Subjects and Methods

The subjects for the study were 32 male and 27 female selected regional players from local juvenile and adult teams. Age, height, and weight data for these groups are summarized in Table 1.

For each group of subjects, we estimated the percentage of body fat and lean body tissue on the basis of four skinfold measurements, according to Durning and Womersley (1974). Maximum oxygen consumption was measured during exhaustive exercises of at least 3 min. duration, which immediately followed three submaximal exercises of 4 min. each. The submaximal exercises were equivalent to 300, 450, and 600 kgm/min for females and 300, 600, and 900 kgm/min for males. All exercises were performed on a Monark friction bicycle/ergometer, at a pedaling speed of 50 rpm. Oxygen consumption was determined by the open circuit method, in which the expired air was collected in a Tissot spirometer and later analyzed in a Schölander apparatus.

The $\dot{V}_{O_2}$ max was estimated in a number of ways. One estimation was based on data from the second submaximal workload and its respective cardiac frequency, using the Astrand and Ryhming Nomogram (1954). A second estimation was based on physical work capacity 170 (PWC 170) and on the equation proposed by Knuttgen (1967), where PWC 170 was obtained by interpolation or extrapolation. Finally, $\dot{V}_{O_2}$ max was calculated through equations proposed by Shephard (1970), using the $\dot{V}_{O_2}$ of submaximal exercise, by Fox (1973), using the PWC 150 calculated according to the ergometric method of Balke (Pini, 1978) to estimate $\dot{V}_{O_2}$ max, and by Von Dobeln et al. (1967) formula.

Oxygen consumption was calculated indirectly using the step-test of Margaria (1965) and Balke (Pini, 1978) and the field test based on races of 12 and 15 min. The results of the 12-min. race were expressed in terms of $\dot{V}_{O_2}$ max according to the equations proposed by Balke (1963) and Cooper (1968), and the results of the 15-min. race were expressed as $\dot{V}_{O_2}$ max according to the equation of Batista (Pini, 1978).

Maximum anaerobic capacity was determined according to the Wingate Anaerobic Test method proposed by Bar-Or (1978); the level of physical preparation was evaluated according to the physical test and the Volley Index, as recommended by the training commission of the International Federation of Volleyball (IFVB).

Results

Data on height, weight, percentage of body fat, and percentage of lean body tissue for the four groups are summarized in Table 1.

Table 1—Mean Values and Standard Deviations for
Physical and Physiological Variables in 57 Regional Select Chilean Volleyball Players

	Female		Male	
	Juveniles (n = 16)	Adults (n = 9)	Juveniles (n = 20)	Adults (n = 12)
Age (years)	15.69 ± 0.77	19.63 ± 1.65	16.25 ± 0.69	21.50 ± 2.69
Height (cm)	160 ± 7	163 ± 3	175 ± 7	179 ± 7
Weight (kg)	55.78 ± 6.81	62.08 ± 5.81	65.68 ± 7.87	70.73 ± 5.33
Percentage of fat	13.93 ± 2.51	13.39 ± 2.77	10.41 ± 2.49	11.12 ± 2.22
Lean body weight (kg)	47.36 ± 6.16	52.32 ± 3.51	60.06 ± 8.29	63.48 ± 4.78
$\dot{V}_{O_2}$ max l/min.	2.43 ± 0.34	2.65 ± 0.36	2.97 ± 9.33	4.03 ± 0.47
$\dot{V}_{O_2}$ max ml/kg/min.	44.49 ± 9.82	43.75 ± 10.22	47.30 ± 2.5	67.16 ± 7.50
$\dot{V}_E$ max l/min.	115.58 ± 20.73	126.12 ± 27.90	141.26 ± 30.16	149.67 ± 24.07
HR max (min.)	198 ± 11.59	189 ± 5.98	196 ± 7.59	186 ± 9.58
PWC_{170} (kgm/min.)	694.47 ± 132.66	868.31 ± 188.41	813.83 ± 124.20	1248.74 ± 125.44
Volley index	19.58 ± 14.42	37.20 ± 9.57	57.99 ± 25.35	70.70 ± 25.33
Max anaerobic cap. kgm/5 sec.	197.65 ± 37.69	276.09 ± 55.37	337.68 ± 41.65	379.90 ± 48.24

Females exhibited a higher percentage of body fat than that of males, with a correspondingly lower percentage of lean body tissue.

The variables measured during the exhaustive exercise are summarized in Table 1. The $\dot{V}_{O_2}$ max was significantly higher among males than among females.

Maximum ventilation ($\dot{V}_E$ max), which in most cases was greater than 2 liters/min per kilogram of body weight, and maximum cardiac frequency are standard indicators of exhaustive work loads. In our subjects, the values for cardiac frequency were below the norms for their age groups, which could be interpreted as an effect of training.

The estimation of $\dot{V}_{O_2}$ max by the various methods and equations correlated well with results obtained by the direct method (Table 2).

The values for the Volley Index and maximum anaerobic capacity are summarized in Table 1. The correlation between the Volley Index and $\dot{V}_{O_2}$ max was poor ($r = 0.17$) whereas the correlation between Volley Index and the maximum anaerobic capacity was good ($r = 0.53$).

The anaerobic potential determined through Wingate's Anaerobic Test is summarized in Figure 1.

Discussion

Recently Dal Monte (1979) classified volleyball as a sport of alternating aerobic-anaerobic activities, in which cardiac frequency and oxygen consumption change according to the competitive and tactical situation. This means that the sport falls into the same category as basketball, football, handball, tennis, and ice hockey.

In the groups studied, height and weight were similar to the values for countries with well-developed programs of volleyball (Table 3). This suggests that, from a structural point of view, our subjects should be capable of adapting themselves to the demands of the sport. The proportion of body fat in our volleyball players is higher than that reported both for foreign athletes in general (Belinka, 1972; Di Prampero et al., 1970; Malhotra et al., 1972) and for foreign volleyball players in particular (DeRose, 1973; Williams et al., 1973; Zelenka et al., 1967). This means that our players are carrying additional weight which detracts from their athletic performance. Aerobic potential, anaerobic potential, and the Volley Index have been determined as principal indices of physical aptitude for volleyball. The values for $\dot{V}_{O_2}$ max in our adult players corresponded to those reported for other elite adult players (Table 3). Values for our adult males are similar to those published by Parmet et al. (1975) and Cumming (1970), and our adult females exhibited a potential higher than that found by Kiss et al. (1973). Our

Table 2—Coefficients of Correlation (r)
Between Measured and Estimated Values of $\dot{V}_{O_2}$ Max

Method	Females	Females	Males	Males
12-min. race (Cooper)	0.79	0.82	0.84	0.86
12-min. race (Balke)	0.80	0.81	0.85	0.86
15-min. race (Batista)	0.61	0.63	0.78	0.61
ST[a] (Nomogram A-R)[b]	0.42	0.66	0.41	0.36
ST[a] (Balke)	0.65	0.67	0.61	0.85
ST[a] (Margaria)	0.45	0.53	0.41	0.42
Ergometric bicycle (Balke)	0.88	0.58	0.71	0.89
Ergometric bicycle (nomogram A-R)[b]	0.94	0.96	0.76	0.84
Shephard	0.94	0.91	0.82	0.75
Fox	0.52	0.49	0.57	0.82
Knuttgen	0.95	0.92	0.84	0.95
Von Dobeln et al.	0.51	0.92	0.68	0.71

Note. [a]ST = Step-test; [b]AR = Astrand and Ryhming.

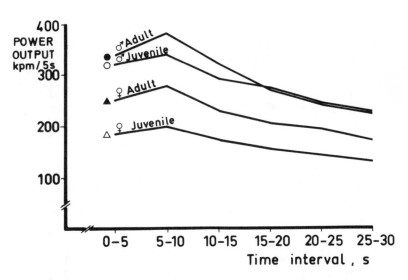

Figure 1—Anaerobic potential according to the Wingate Anaerobic Test method.
△ Juvenile Female Category
▲ Adult Female Category
o Juvenile Male Category
● Adult Male Category

Table 3—Physical Characteristics and Work Capacity of Volleyball Players in Different Studies

Country	N	Sex	Age (years)	Height (cm)	Weight (kg)	Percentage of fat %	Exercise	$\dot{V}_{O_2}$ Max Ml/kg/mn	HR Max (/m)	Author
Brazil	19	F	14.50	165.4	58.50	—	SMBE	33.00	—	Kiss et al. (1973)
Japan	—	F	—	168.1	63.30	—			—	Hukuda and Ishiko (1966)
Chile	16	M	15.69	160.0	55.78	13.93	BE	44.49	198.0	P. Study
Chile	9	M	19.63	163.0	62.08	13.39	BE	43.75	189.0	P. Study
Brazil	35	M	—	176.0	74.40	10.20	—	—	—	De Rose (1973)
Czechoslovakia	12	M	—	178.8	72.50	11.60	—	—	—	Zelenka et al. (1967)
Germany (Frg)	14	M	—	178.5	77.60	—	—	—	—	Hollmann et al. (1962)
UK	9	M	—	174.6	69.40	12.40	—	—	—	Williams et al. (1973)
USA	17	M	—	176.0	70.60	9.90	—	—	—	Serfas (1971)
Canada	6	M	—	—	—	—	B.	51.90	—	Cumming (1970)
USSR	12	M	20.8±07	—	80.20	—	—	56.40	183.2	Parnat et al. (1975)
Chile	20	M	16.25	175.0	65.58	10.41	BE	47.30	196.0	P. Study
Chile	12	M	21.50	179.0	70.73	11.12	BE	57.16	186.0	P. Study

Note. SM = Submaximal; BE = Bicycle ergometer.

values for young males are low, but this could be expected, inasmuch as that group had not yet completed its development. Although it is true that our values for older males correspond to those cited for other adult volleyball players, such is not the case for adult athletes of other aerobic-anaerobic sports, for the data of Williams (1973), DeRose (1973), and Serfass (1971) exceed our own values. With respect to the $\dot{V}_{O_2}$ max, it is worthwhile mentioning the good correlations obtained with the nomogram of Astrand and Rhyming (1954) in the bicycle ergometric test, with the formulas of Fox (1973) and Knuttgen (1967), and with the 12-min. track race. The latter is easily applied and low cost and could be easily utilized to obtain indices of aerobic potential, as long as the subjects are highly motivated.

The Volley Index values reported in this study are inferior to those reported for countries with a more highly developed program of volleyball, according to the data of Kato (1978). Values for selected female student players in Japan and Peru were higher than those for our young females (74.30 and 78.10), and values for selected male students and university players in Japan also exceed those for our young males (104.60 and 112.10). Such inferiority suggests a poor conditioning of our volleyball players, with respect to the height and jumping potential equivalent. It is known that the human organism adapts to growing demands imposed on its physical capacity by improving with respect to the group of factors which determine such capacity. Through this adaptive process, systematic physical activity and sports develop the physical capacity of the subject. Given this, our results suggest that from a structural point of view, and using physiological condition as a base, our subjects suffer from no particular disadvantages. Given the opportunity for adequate athletic training, they could obtain higher levels of fitness. The lower levels of fitness we found could be explained by the lack of an efficient training technique or by inappropriate methods of training.

With this knowledge of these variations in our athletic population, we can establish a more adequate training program to obtain a maximum of fitness, without compromising the development and health of the subjects.

References

Astrand, P.O. 1976. Quantification of exercise capability and evaluation of physical capacity in man. *Progress Cardior. Diseases* **19**:51-70.

Astrand, P.O., and Rodahl, K. 1970. *Textbook of Work Physiology.* International student edition. McGraw-Hill Book Co. Kogokusha Ltd, Japan.

Astrand, P.O., and Ryhming, J. 1954. Nomogram for calculation of aerobic capacity (physical fitness) from pulse rate during submaximal work. *J. Appl.*

Physiol. **7**:218-221.

Balke, B. 1963. A simple field test for assessment of physical fitness. Federal Aviation Agency, Oklahoma City, OK, cited by Godoy and Quintana, 1978. Estimacion del consumo maximo de oxigeno mediante la carrera de 12 minutos (Estimation of maximum oxygen consumption using the 12 minute track race.) *Arch. Soc. Chil. Med. Dep.* **23**:10-13 (September).

Bar-Or, O. 1978. A new anaerobic capacity test. Characteristics and applications. Paper presented at the 21st World Congress in Sports Medicine, Brasilia, September 7-12.

Behnke, A.R., Feen, B.G., and Weltham, W.C. 1942. The specific gravity of healthy men. *J. Amer. Med. Ass.* **118**:495-501.

Cooper, K.H. 1968. A means of assessing maximal oxygen intake: Correlation between field and treadmill testing. *JAMA* **203**:201-204.

Cumming, G.R. 1970. Fitness testing of athletes. *Can. Fam. Physician,* August pp. 48-52.

Dal Monte, 1979. Clasificacion fisiologica de las actividades de portivas y funcion cardiovascular (Physiological classification of athletic activities and cardiovascular function.) *Arch. Soc. Chile,* Med. Dep. **23**:2.

DeRose, H. 1973. O exame medico do jogador de futebol (The medical examination for soccer players.) *Med do Esporte* **1**:15-21

Di Prampero, P.E., Limas, F.P., and Sasai, G. 1970. Maximal muscular power, aerobic and anaerobic, in 116 athletes performing at the XIX Olympic Games in Mexico. *Ergonomics* **13**:665-674.

Donoso, H., and Godoy, J.D. 1977. Capacidad fisica en futbolistas profesionales chilenos (Physical capacity in professional Chilean soccer players.) *Arch. Soc. Chil Med. Dep.* **22**(dic. 77) 17-20.

Durning, J.V.G.A., and Womersley, J. 1974. Body fat assessed from total body density and its estimation from skinfold thickness: Measurements on 481 men and women aged from 16-72 years. *Br. Nutr.* **32**:77-97.

Fox, E. 1973. A simple, accurate technique for predicting maximal aerobic power. *J. Appl. Physiol.* **35**:914-916.

Hukuda, K., and Ishiko, T. 1966. Comparison between physical fitness of Japanese and European athletes. In: K. Kato (ed.), *Proceedings of International Congress of Sport Sciences,* 1964. Japanese Union of Sport Sciences, Tokyo.

Kato, A. 1978. La prepacion fisica en la evolucion del voleybol (Physical preparation in the evolution of volleyball.) *Deporte y Recreacion-Chile,* August 1978.

Kiss, M.A., Rocha-erreira, M.B., Souza, P., Vasconcelos, R.M., Santos, F., Anzai, K., Pagan, J., Andre, J., Rodriguez, R., Bosco, J., Baccrala, L.T., and Pini, M.C. 1973. Potencia maxima aerobica en atletas de selecos Paulistas e Brasileiras. (Maximum aerobic potential in selected athletes from Sao Paulo and Brazil.) *Med. Esporte* :23-30.

Knuttgen, H. 1967, Aerobic capacity of adolescents. *J. Appl. Physiol.* **22**:655-658.

Malhotra, M.S., Ramaswamy, S.S., Joseph, H.T., and Gupta, J.S. 1972. Functional capacity and body composition in different classes of Indian athletes. *Ind. J. Physiol. Pharm.* **16**:301-316.

Margaria, R., Aghemo, P., and Rovelli, E. 1965. Indirect determination of maximal oxygen consumption in man. *J. Appl. Physiol* **20**:1070-1073.

Parnat, J., Viru, A., Savi, T., and Nurmekivi, A. Indices of aerobic work capacity and cardio-vascular responses during exercises in athletes specializing in different events. *J. Sport Med. Phys. Fitness* **15**:100-105.

Pini, M.C. 1978. Fisiologia Sportiva. (Sport Physiology.) Guanabara Koagan S.A., Rio de Janeiro.

Serfass, R.C. 1971. Changes in cardiorespiratory fitness and body composition of participants in selected physical education classes. Ph.D. dissertation, University of Minnesota. Cited by Kollias, J., Buskirk, E.R., Howley, E.T., and Loomis, J.L. 1972. Cardiorespiratory and body composition measurement of high school football players. *Res. Quart.* **43**:472-478.

Shephard, R.J. 1970. Computer programs for solution of the Astrand nomogram and the calculation of body surface area. *J. Sports Med.* **10**:206-210.

Von Dobeln, W., Astrand, I., and Bergstrom, A. 1967. An analysis of age and other factors related to maximal oxygen uptake. *J. Appl. Physiol.* **22**:934-938.

Williams, C., Reid, R.M., and Coutts, R. 1973. Observation on the aerobic power of university rugby players and professional soccer players. *Brit. J. Sports Med.* **7**:390-391.

Zelenka, V., Seliger, V., and Ondrey, O. 1967. Specific function testing of young football players. *J. Sports Med. Phys. Fitness* **7**:143-147.